# At Wit's End

# At Wit's End

Plain Talk on Alzheimer's for Families and Clinicians
Second Edition

George Kraus, Ph.D.

Purdue University Press
West Lafayette, Indiana

Library of Congress Cataloging-in-Publication Data

Names: Kraus, George, 1950- author.
Title: At wit's end : plain talk on Alzheimer's for families and clinicians /
    George Kraus, Ph.D.
Description: Second edition. | West Lafayette, Indiana : Purdue University
    Press, [2017] | Includes bibliographical references and index.
Identifiers: LCCN 2016016854| ISBN 9781557537676 (pbk. : alk. paper) | ISBN
    9781612494708 (epdf) | ISBN 9781612494715 (epub)
Subjects:  LCSH: Alzheimer's disease.
Classification: LCC RC523 .K736 2017 | DDC 616.8/31—dc23
LC record available at https://lccn.loc.gov/2016016854

*Cover image from CelsoDiniz/iStock/Thinkstock*

*I dedicate this book to my beautiful and inspirational wife, Lori.*

*I love you deeply, my friend.*

# Contents

# Acknowledgments

Creating a book like this takes support, guidance, and a little inspiration, and I am so grateful for all the help I've received. To all of my friends, colleagues, and family, thank you. You have contributed more than you know to this book and to my life.

It's a rare thing to find the kindness you want to give others reflected in someone else. To John Chang, Ph.D., of Wright State University—for providing me those many hours of consultation on the psychology of the elderly. The time we spent together was essential in developing my practice specialty as a geropsychologist. Your clinical expertise, friendship, and support have helped me set a sound foundation for my clinical work with Alzheimer's patients.

Over the years that I have provided care and consulted to Livingston Care Center, I have worked with some incredible people—Samuel Berger, Sharon Clay, Hilda Claypool, Brenda Cooper, Kara Crutcher, Jennifer Foley, Patty Free, Cynthia Gifford, Haitham Imam, Romona Pollard, Linda Riebe, Kim Schooler, Rischell Snow, Debbie Steward, Lynn Thurston, Vladimir Trakhter, Dale Valiquette, Barb Vocke, Amy Walters, and Luther Wright III—thank you all for making me feel so welcome and appreciated. The stable center of my work there, though, has been Julie Upchurch, LSW, Director of Social Services, and two of her very finest assistants, Casandra Watson and Bo Hobbs—I am so very grateful for all your efforts in supporting my connection with your residents and making the time I've spent at Livingston meaningful and fun. Finally, I want to offer my heartfelt gratitude to Bil Ferrar, Director of Social Services, of Patriot Ridge Community for your dedication and commitment to your residents there, and especially to Ann Wilder, Director of Activities, and Jackie Davis of Patriot Ridge Community—thank you both for the fine activities programming you've offered there. I also want to thank Jennifer Jenkins and

Sue Holston of Tampico Terrace Care Center; Lydia Swagerty and Trisha Oliver of Rheem Valley Convalescent Hospital; and Sue Fordon and Karen Barnes-Jarvis of Hospice of the East Bay for all their help and support in welcoming and integrating me into my new California community.

To all the clinicians and staff of Layh and Associates of Yellow Springs, Ohio—Joyce Appell, LPC, Bruce Heckman, Ph.D., Casey Kelliher, Psy.D., Jim Kane, LPC, Lorena Kvalheim, Psy.D., Melissa Layman-Guadalupe, Ph.D., Kate LeVesconte, Psy.D., Kathi Lewis, Psy.D., Angela Branch, Katie Malone, and Ruth Willfong—thanks for all the valuable help, feedback, and support you have offered me over the years. And I'd like to give a special thanks to Jack Layh, Ph.D., your experience and indispensable assistance have been invaluable in helping me develop my practice as a psychologist.

To all the wonderful staff at the Greene County Libraries of Yellow Springs, Ohio—Connie Collett, Alan, Staiger, Rick Mickels, Pat Siemer, Peggy Townshend, Tricia Gelmini, Paul Cooper, Lyn Bobo—thanks for all the help and technical guidance in maneuvering through your world of information science, and especially to Amy Margolin of the Greene County Library of Xenia for tracking down the sea of interlibrary loan items I requested.

To all my colleagues at Midwest Behavioral Care of Dayton, Ohio—Steve Pearce, Psy.D., Deb Sowald, Psy.D., Phyllis Kuehnl-Walters, Ph.D., Gary Dixon, LISW, and Lee Wolfe, LPCC—your support and good advice helped me in so many ways to develop my practice and skills as a clinician. I want to thank Tina Bowers, Ruth Waymire, and especially Jennifer Shank and Tabby Masters for all the encouragement and fun you brought into my life working there as I wrote this book.

I want to thank David Goldberg, M.D., of Greene Memorial Hospital—I really appreciated the support and encouragement you gave me when I first presented the seeds for this book at my Grand Rounds talk on dementia.

To Ed Klein, Ph.D., and Walt Stone, M.D., of the University of Cincinnati, thank you for all the sound academic advice, clinical pearls, and kind truths you gave me during my post-doctoral clinical training. You are two of my wise mentors, and it was such a gift to have been able to work with you.

To Gary Gemmill, Ph.D., and Celeste Sinton, M.D., mentors and emotional guides both—thanks for teaching me just how much I can enjoy learning about my vulnerabilities and trusting myself. You each have brought me so much wisdom and faith in the process, and I will forever be grateful to you both.

To my Uncle Chick—although you have long passed, I want to thank you so much for helping me begin to really see and like myself in ways I never had.

Your book with Maxwell Maltz and that summer workshop, "How to Live and Be Free Through Psychocybernetics," inspired me to pursue my passion for psychology. And to Aunt Shirley, thank you so much for all the loving guidance you have given me.

To my sisters, Pat and Betty—your encouragement and love has been a silent undercurrent in all of my efforts here. Thank you, Pat, for your insightful suggestions and Betty, for your simple and beautiful artwork in the book. And to my parents—somewhere you are watching from above, reading this, and smiling with joy.

To my Aunt Peggy, our family historian—your love and encyclopedic knowledge of the genealogy of all the clinicians in our family has contributed to a strong sense of professional identity and connectedness to the traditions of my past. Your love and support have quietly helped me believe in myself.

To Tom Tuttle and Sandy Novak, thank you both for all your incredible insights and optimism. Your experience and wisdom made finding a publisher exciting and fun. And to Vivian Tuttle, my wonderful new mom, thanks for reviewing an early draft of the book and for all the love and silliness you bring into my life. It's great being in your family.

To my wife, Lori, and to all the special children in my life—Aurianna, Michael, Nancy, Nathan, Miles, Dee, and Axs—you have brightened my life in ways that go beyond words. I love you all very much.

To the late Margaret Hunt of Purdue University Press, thank you for all your editorial wisdom, patience, and faith in making *At Wit's End* (2006) the very best it could be. I also want to thank Katherine Purple and Peter Froehlich for shepherding this new and updated edition along its way and Kelley Kimm, Bryan Shaffer, and Mary Beth Deitz for their invaluable assistance in this process.

To Jennifer Moye, Ph.D., ABPP, from VA Boston and Harvard Medical School, your editing suggestions were invaluable in making the second edition of *At Wit's End* the very best it could be.

And finally, to all my elderly patients, who have taught me about the courage and dignity of living with Alzheimer's. I feel a great deal of indebtedness to you—for the time you spent with me, for the courage you showed me, and for the wisdom you revealed to me.

# Preface

> "The soul comes to the end of its long
> journey and naked and alone draws near
> to the divine."[1]

To first hear that your mother or father or anyone you love has Alzheimer's leaves an empty feeling in the pit of your stomach. There are over 5 million families in the United States who have received just this kind of news, and I don't think very many of them have really known quite what to do with it. It's very difficult to have a family member or a close friend suffer from an incurable disease. It's hard to know just what to say sometimes, how to help them, how to be with them. For those who know someone with Alzheimer's, this is no exception.

What helps, though, is being willing to risk getting close enough to them to really understand what it means to have Alzheimer's. This takes courage. But if we are willing to do this we make ourselves more available to the person—we can walk in his shoes, and in doing so, we open ourselves to the possibility of discovering those precious and intimate moments of closeness and connectedness that make our lives truly meaningful. It also makes the help we give that much more effective. With this in mind, I would like to take you on a journey of discovery about Alzheimer's—to help you get really close to it—to help you learn about the impact Alzheimer's has on those who suffer from it and the effect it has on families, caregivers, and ourselves.

From a physical point of view, Alzheimer's is a disease characterized by the destruction and degeneration of tissue in the brain. Its toll on the human spirit, however, is even more devastating. Alzheimer's slowly robs its hosts of their memory, their ability to think, and ultimately, the very sense of their own existence. Alzheimer's is a disease for which there is no cure—only medicines that can slow the progression of its symptoms or postpone its inevitable conclusion. This point of view is well known. From another perspective, however, Alzheimer's is a psychiatric disorder—a mental illness—one that triggers a wide array of emotional and behavioral problems. These types of problems can be treated with medicines, but they can also be treated with counseling and psychotherapy, and this perspective is much less well known.

Counseling people with Alzheimer's? Can you do that? For many Alzheimer's patients, the answer is an emphatic "Yes!" Understanding Alzheimer's from a psychological model (and not strictly from a medical one) opens up possibilities for new and expanded ways of relating to those afflicted with this illness. New intervention possibilities like these are not only available to the professional and paraprofessional care provider, but they are also available to family members, friends, or anyone who provides care for someone with this disorder. Everyone in the individual's family and social support system can learn to communicate better with the Alzheimer's sufferer. It takes knowledge and understanding and being able to identify and relate to the problems of Alzheimer's as they arise.

Making the distinction between Alzheimer's as a medical illness and Alzheimer's as a mental disorder is essential. From a medical perspective, Alzheimer's is a *disease,* like cancer, heart disease, or emphysema. As a disease, it progresses, its symptoms worsen, and eventually, it's fatal. Alzheimer's as a disease implies that it is a medical problem with medical solutions. Increasingly, we hear of "breakthrough research" on the genetic and biochemical links with Alzheimer's. We also hear announcements of new image-scanning methods to better identify the illness or new drugs to treat its accelerating symptoms. These discoveries are important, but regarding what is known and generally applied in the treatment of Alzheimer's, its treatment has essentially been relegated to medical staff prescribing and recommending medical interventions.

In addition to being classified as a medical illness, though, Alzheimer's is a *mental illness,* just like schizophrenia, depression, or anxiety disorder.[2] Alzheimer's as a mental disorder implies, however, that in addition to medical interventions, there are also psychiatric and psychological treatment interventions available. In addition to high-tech detection methods and new medicines to treat the spread of the disease, the symptoms of Alzheimer's can also be treated through psychological methods that include individual counseling, group interventions, interventions designed to change the person's physical surroundings, and through medicines and educational strategies to improve the person's ability to cope with the emotional distress and cognitive loss. This is the focus of *At Wit's End*. This book is intended to be a simple, straightforward, and easy-to-read summary of what is currently known about this devastating disorder, as free as possible from technical jargon and impractical detail.

About one in three of us will eventually provide care for someone with Alzheimer's. Given the tremendous amount of care required to safeguard the medical well-being and mental health stability of people with Alzheimer's, *At Wit's End* is intended to offer new options for clinicians, family members, and the many other caregivers who assist, support, and help to ease the impact of this quiet killer. The stress of providing care to a person with Alzheimer's can be considerable, but caring for someone with Alzheimer's can also be extremely rewarding. I have talked with many care providers whose pride in what they are doing far outweighs the challenges with which they struggle. For me, it's been the joy of helping Alzheimer's sufferers and their families hold on to the value they place on living. *At Wit's End* has been written to enhance your knowledge about the psychiatric and psychological aspects of Alzheimer's as it helps you discover a wealth of effective interventions too infrequently utilized.

There are many excellent books on Alzheimer's—ones that address the medical, financial, legal, and daily care needs of those afflicted with the disease. There are excellent sources of information on a variety of issues related to managing guardianship, powers of attorney, living wills, life and health-care insurance, and on making choices about assisted-living facilities, nursing homes, in-home care, and safety preparation of the person's living environment. These are all important areas of concern, and I have tried to provide a wealth of references to help you learn more about them. There has also been a great deal written about the self-preservation needs of family members and other caregivers who have been left with the disheartening and often daunting task of managing the afflicted person's waning competencies. References to these excellent sources of information are also included.

The thrust of *At Wit's End*, however, is on the psychological life of the Alzheimer's sufferer. It focuses on the whole person and his social, psychological, emotional, physical, and spiritual life. *Part 1: What Is Alzheimer's?* covers the basics of the disorder, how it can be distinguished from normal aging, and how it is similar to and different from other medical conditions that mimic its symptoms. *Part 2: How to Evaluate for Alzheimer's* deals with a variety of assessment methods that are commonly used to gauge the extent and progression of the disease. These include methods of measuring how the disorder affects changes in functional abilities and how the issue of competence to complete tasks of daily living is viewed by the psychiatric and legal communities.

*Part 3: Disturbances in Mood and Perception* covers the array of emotional and behavioral problems frequently encountered in Alzheimer's—things like anxiety and agitation, depression, anger and impatience, inappropriate expressions of sexuality, wandering, and other troubling behavioral conditions. In this section, special attention is given to the issue of geriatric depression and its reciprocal relationship with Alzheimer's. Also examined in this section is how Alzheimer's affects distortions in rational thinking and psychotic disturbances in sensory perceptions. Finally, in *Part 4: Medical and Psychological Treatment Approaches,* I discuss traditional and alternative medicines that are available to treat the disease itself and the emotional and intellectual symptoms commonly stemming from the disorder. I also discuss changes that can be made to the afflicted person's physical surroundings, simple and commonsense ways of enhancing communication, new ways of improving coping abilities, fun learning activities useful in stimulating and maintaining the afflicted person's thinking and emotional stability, and finally, ways of preventing the disease.

My hope is that reading this book will be just the beginning of your continued learning about Alzheimer's. The more you know and share about Alzheimer's as a medical illness and as a mental health disorder, the more the suffering from this devastating disease can be abated.

# Second Edition Introduction

Over the last ten years since *At Wit's End* was published, there have been many promising new treatments touted but not delivered. Nevertheless, every week seems to bring new research to light on the causes and possible cures for Alzheimer's disease. There have been many dashed hopes for unraveling the mysteries of Alzheimer's, but social science and medical research continue unabated. Their spirit and determination keep us going, and for this, the world and I are grateful.

The other night, I was watching *The Green Mile*—a film that, for me, never fails to impress. Tom Hanks plays the lead role as Paul Edgecomb, a prison officer in charge of death row, and at the end of the film Paul reflects back on his life and the path he has traveled, saying, "We each owe a death—there are no exceptions . . . but, oh God, sometimes the Green Mile seems so long." This is a universal truth—one for all of us—and especially for those with Alzheimer's.

Heart disease and cancer are the leading causes of death in the United States, but dementia is the third. Although dementia covers a broad array of illnesses, the most common is Alzheimer's, and this illness is as important a topic today as it has ever been. It's important from a medical perspective, from a family and social perspective, and from the point of view of our evolving culture. It has been found that without a psychological test for dementia, the patient, the physician, and family members are all unaware of the presence of it in 40–70 percent of the cases. It has also been found that while 80 percent of geriatric physicians and geriatric psychiatrists saw benefits to disclosing a dementia diagnosis to their patients, only 40 percent consistently did so.[1] Additionally, it has been found that an Alzheimer's patient in the last five years of life incurs medical costs of almost $300,000. Compare that to the cost incurred by patients with heart disease—which is about $175,000—or by patients with cancer—which is about $173,000. The more alarming fact is that those with Medicare received about $100,000 from that insurer, but the rest of the costs were paid by either secondary insurers *or by the patients and their families.*[2] It is estimated that in 2015, $226 billion was spent in the United States in the fight against Alzheimer's. Finding a cure is vital.

Having worked with older adults in my outpatient practice and in nursing homes for many years, I understand that there is no single issue facing us more universally than the inevitability of aging. Life expectancies are extending at rates never before seen. (Recent reports claim that a Kazakhstani woman named Sahan Dosova lived to be 130.) And while we will be more likely to develop dementia as we age still further, we also have the chance to live longer and more meaningful lives. This is why in 2006 I wrote *At Wit's End,* and this is why I am offering an update on this important topic. I hope you find it helpful, and I hope you find it comforting.

# Part 1

# What Is Alzheimer's?

# 1

# The Basics

"Everything that has a beginning has an ending. Make your peace with that and all will be well."[1]

When I was a boy, there was a very old man down the street who sometimes walked in our neighborhood in his pajamas. Many of the neighbors thought he was crazy, but we really just wondered what was wrong with him. Everybody used to say, "He's just old!" When I was ten my Grampa Ike came to live with us. Sometimes, he thought he was in the bathroom and would pee down the laundry chute. My mother used to explain to me, "People do that when they get old." For many years, that's just what I believed. But as I wound up learning much later in life, these problems are signs of disease and not a natural stage of old age.

Contrary to popular belief, senility (the loss of memory and thinking ability in late life) is not a natural stage of a person's development. As we age, we all suffer predictable impairments in our physical well-being. We get colder, shorter, weaker, and we can't think quite as fast. These are natural processes that I will discuss further in chapter 2. For now, though, it's important to emphasize that Alzheimer's is a disease and not a natural part of our aging process.

## What Are My Chances of Getting Alzheimer's Disease?

Every few years my parents would go to the race track to see the trotters run. They would usually play the favorites, but occasionally my father would smile, showing us his winning ticket to a 10 to 1 long shot he'd bet. Those are about the average odds of getting Alzheimer's: 1 in 10.

According to the American Psychiatric Association, approximately 1 in 40 Americans over the age of 60 suffers from Alzheimer's dementia. This is an estimate of severe cases only. When moderately severe cases of Alzheimer's are considered, the rate increases to about 3 in 40. Include mild cases in the statistic, and the prevalence rate rises to 4 in 40. This translates to about 350,000 new cases of Alzheimer's each year in the United States. There are currently over 5 million people in the United States with Alzheimer's, and estimates are that the number of cases will quadruple in the next 20 years. People with mild to moderate Alzheimer's live from 2 to 10 years with the illness; people with severe Alzheimer's live from 1 to 5 years.

Depending on the age when symptoms begin to appear, there are two classifications of Alzheimer's disease: *early-onset* Alzheimer's, also known as familial Alzheimer's (age 65 or younger) and *late-onset* Alzheimer's (after age 65). Only about 5 percent of all the cases of Alzheimer's occur before the age of 65. Although extremely rare, the youngest known patient with Alzheimer's was 28 years old. For those 60–65 years old, the prevalence of the disease in the general population is about 1 percent. The frequency of its occurrence then doubles every 5 years thereafter—that is, for those 65–70, the likelihood of developing the disease is about 2 percent; for those 70–75, it's about 4 percent, and so on. People who are over 80 years old have about a 1 in 6 chance of getting the disease, and for those adults who live to be 85, there is a one-in-three chance they will get Alzheimer's. From the time the disease is first diagnosed, the average length of survival for late-onset Alzheimer's is about 8 to 10 years. Early-onset Alzheimer's progresses faster, and the average length of survival for this type of Alzheimer's is 6 to 8 years. President Ronald Reagan was diagnosed in November 1992 when he was 81; he died in June 2004 when he was 93. Early-onset Alzheimer's may be in the making for some 20 years or more before symptoms first appear.

Our population is aging, skilled services for Alzheimer's sufferers are dwindling, and the cost to care for them is rising. Approximately 75,000 people in this country will turn 100 years old this year. By the year 2050, there will be 800,000 more Americans each year turning 100,[2] and it is projected that by then there will be 10 million people with Alzheimer's in the country. The latest government statistics show that there are currently about 16,000 certified nursing facilities in the United States that serve people with Alzheimer's and other dementias, but the number of facilities has been falling steadily since 1998.[3] About half of all Alzheimer's sufferers, though, receive their care at home. Of those who live at home, many report, however, that it often takes on a strange and unfamiliar feel to it—like living in a motel.[4] Alzheimer's is a serious public health issue that is estimated to have cost Americans over $200 billion last year. The cost to an Alzheimer's family is about $60,000 per year. All this is to say that as our population gets older, it becomes more and more important to understand who gets Alzheimer's disease, when they might get it, and what can be done about it.

**What Are the Risk Factors?**

My father died of a heart attack—his fourth. I wonder sometimes if the same thing will happen to me. I know, though, that if I eat healthy foods, exercise, and watch my cholesterol I will lower my chances of dying from a heart attack. Alzheimer's has its risk factors, too.

The most prominent risk factors for Alzheimer's are having a history of family members with the disease, having incurred a head injury, and having little education. About half the people with a family history of the disease develop Alzheimer's by age 80–90. Head injuries also make it more likely that the disease will develop. Curiously, low education appears to correlate with the diagnosis. Researchers have speculated that this is true, because people who have more education may be more articulate or witty and may be better able to mask or shift attention away from others noticing signs of the disease.

Ethnic background also seems to play a role in the development of the disease. Research on ethnic differences in Alzheimer's has been ongoing, but studies show that African Americans are nearly twice as likely as whites to develop the disorder.[5] It has also been found that Hispanic Americans are about one and one-half times more likely to develop the illness than whites.[6]

The reason for these differences is not entirely clear but might be explained by ethnic differences in overall longevity. Demographic research on the elderly has shown that African Americans live to be about 75 years old; Native Americans, about 77 years old; whites live to be about 79 years old; Hispanic Americans live to be about 83 years old; and Asian Americans live to be about 87 years old.[7] What this implies is that while we might imagine "old age" for whites beginning at age 65, this is lower for some ethnic minorities.

Depression also may be a risk factor for Alzheimer's. Of those who have a major depressive episode in their lifetime, about two-thirds have it before they are 50. About another one-third, however, will have it in their 60s, and of those who have their first episode in their 60s, it is more likely that they will develop Alzheimer's than those who have their first episode earlier in life. Because depression is also a risk factor for heart attacks, stroke, and diabetes, just how significant this statistic will turn out to be is yet unclear.[8]

Researchers are also paying more attention to the early and more subtle signs of Alzheimer's—what has been called *mild cognitive impairment* (MCI), a condition similar to Alzheimer's but less severe. MCI seems to be an important risk factor for Alzheimer's. The symptoms of Alzheimer's and of mild cognitive impairment, however, seem to be recognized by physicians much less than expected. This is so because there are no standardized definitions or measures for MCI. For example, in one study, only 3 percent of bona fide Alzheimer's cases were properly identified by psychiatrists despite the symptoms of Alzheimer's actually being present.[9] Based on other research, as many as 75 percent of people with moderate dementia and 95 percent of people with mild dementia escape timely diagnosis. These are sobering statistics in light of the fact that the conversion rate from mild cognitive impairment to Alzheimer's disease is estimated to be 15–20 percent per year.[10] Figure 1a presents these and other factors believed to increase the risk for Alzheimer's.

Early identification of the illness is vital to effective treatment and extended longevity. It is estimated that a five-year delay in the onset of the disease might decrease the number of people who get the disease by one-half![11] Early detection and treatment are important in several ways. Early treatment helps treat the disease before symptoms become more severe. Treatment at earlier stages also helps ease some of the predictable emotional problems, like depression and worry, that often accompany early signs of the illness. Early detection and treatment also provide the family with additional time and tools to adjust to their loved one's having the disease.[12]

**Figure 1a.** Risk Factors for Alzheimer's Disease

| | |
|---|---|
| ◆ Age | ◆ Low level of physical activity |
| ◆ Alcoholism | ◆ History of smoking |
| ◆ Low education | ◆ Non-stimulating environment |
| ◆ Family history of Alzheimer's | ◆ Presence of mild cognitive |
| ◆ History of head trauma | impairment |
| ◆ Being female | ◆ Low folic acid levels |
| ◆ African-American ethnicity | ◆ Low vitamin $B_{12}$ levels |

## What Causes Alzheimer's?

Is it nature or nurture? Whenever the issue arises about what causes disease we come to this frequently asked question. As with other diseases, the answer with Alzheimer's is "It's both." The illness is influenced by our genetics and biology and it is affected by what happens to us after we are born. Estimates vary wildly about the role of genetics, but research from twin studies has shown that up to 80 percent of Alzheimer's cases may be attributable to genetics.[13]

A great deal of research on what causes Alzheimer's has focused on the genetics and molecular biology of the illness. The research has been based on two principal avenues of investigation: (1) what is referred to as the *amyloid hypothesis* and (2) what is called the *cholinergic hypothesis*. Figure 1b summarizes these two approaches.

The amyloid hypothesis proposes that a protein called beta-amyloid is in high concentration in the areas of the brain where most of the tissue and neural degeneration from Alzheimer's occurs. These beta-amyloid–rich areas are called *amyloid plaques,* and under the microscope, each plaque looks like a sore, where the healthy tissue in the middle has died. Understanding how to

**Figure 1b.** The Two Primary Avenues of Research on Alzheimer's

| | |
|---|---|
| **The Amyloid Hypothesis** proposes that a protein, called beta-amyloid, is in high concentration in the areas of the brain where most of the tissue and neural degeneration from Alzheimer's occurs. These areas are called plaques. | **The Cholinergic Hypothesis** proposes that a deficiency in a chemical called acetylcholine, which helps nerves in the brain communicate with one another, is more likely to be found in people who have Alzheimer's than it is in those who don't. |

better control the level of beta-amyloid in the brain, it has been presumed, will lead to better methods of controlling the progression of the disease.

The cholinergic hypothesis proposes that in people with Alzheimer's, there is a deficiency in a chemical called *acetylcholine,* which helps nerves in the brain communicate with one another. We will discuss acetylcholine and its role in brain functioning in more detail later on. Better understanding of the relationship between acetylcholine and Alzheimer's, scientists believe, will lead to advances in treatment. Pharmaceutical research has been predominantly guided by this hypothesis, and the medicines designed to enhance acetylcholine levels will be discussed in more detail later on in chapter 12.

It's fascinating to me that our genetics and, perhaps, our own natural biology are not exclusive factors, however, in determining whether we get Alzheimer's or exhibit its symptoms. According to theories on brain development, the brain can grow and change in adulthood because of what we do with it. Similar to the way jogging helps build our endurance for other sports, mental cross-training can help build new nerve connections, even late in life, that can fend off the disease. For example, one way we might minimize our chances of suffering from the symptoms of Alzheimer's is by mentally exercising ourselves with new and novel tasks. I will discuss much more about this topic in chapter 15, but here's an example of what I mean. Based on the autobiographies of nuns written some 60 years earlier, it was found that the mental sharpness of these women was greater for those who lived longer. More specifically, the longer a nun lived, the more likely her autobiography contained unusual, multisyllabic words or phrases rich with ideas.[14] Other research has shown that people who regularly read, solve crossword puzzles, play cards or checkers, or visit museums may be less likely to experience mental decline. The conclusion: learning strengthens the brain's resistance to decline. In other words, mental exercise helps!

Recent research has also suggested that the level of education we achieve may somehow protect us from Alzheimer's. Studies have shown that regardless of how elderly they may be, people who graduate from college may be less vulnerable to memory loss than people with only an elementary school education.[15] What this means is that the brain may store capacities in reserve that get released later when needed. Other studies have shown that when highly educated Alzheimer's patients are matched with less educated ones—that is, matched by having symptoms that were comparable in severity—their brain scans revealed that the disease was more advanced in the educated group.[16] Research has shown that the ability of the brain to store capacity in reserve may also be at work in people who do not have Alzheimer's. What's important to understand here is that while genetics and biology obviously play important roles in causing Alzheimer's, what we do with our brain can affect how, or even if, the symptoms of the disease significantly develop.

It's a challenging part of life, perhaps the most challenging, to accept that our lives will eventually end. We might be comforted by the belief in the hereafter or may imagine our spirits becoming part of a larger universe, but for those with Alzheimer's and for all of us who care for them, the task, ultimately, is to make peace with this indisputable fact. If we can do this, our lives and the lives of the people for whom we provide care can become transformed.

# 2

# Normal Aging

"In life, we cannot avoid change. Freedom
and happiness are found in the flexibility
and ease with which we move through
changes."

My hairline is receding. My endurance isn't quite what it used to be. I'm getting hair in places I never did. I'm not worried, though. I'm not rushing off to the doctor about it. That's because I know that it's normal and that eventually everyone will go through these kinds of changes. Normal aging is a natural process. We can't avoid it. So before we talk more about Alzheimer's, let's look at this disease in the context of normal aging.

As we get older, there are certain predictable bodily changes that will occur. These changes are not signs or symptoms of disease but expectable, understandable, and anticipated developments in how we all age. For example, when we can't find our keys or momentarily can't remember someone's name, it doesn't signify that we have a disease. As we get older, there is natural decline. Instead of feeling alarmed when we forget something, most of us just say to ourselves, "That's one of those senior moments," or we brush it off to normal forgetting. Over the years, there have been many terms used for common forgetfulness in later life, but most recently, researchers have called these natural incidents of forgetting age-consistent memory decline.[1] Here's a list of some of the other normal and natural changes we can expect to experience as we advance into old age.[2]

## Appearance
- Our nose and ears will get bigger.
- We will lose height because our bone mass declines. This is especially true in women.
- We'll get colder more easily because we'll have less insulation.

## Mobility
- We'll be less mobile and agile because after age 50 or so our muscles will lose strength, especially in our legs.
- We will be less resistant to stress and fractures because our bones will lose mass and will get more brittle. This is especially true in women.
- Our tendons and ligaments will be more prone to injury because our joints will get weaker.

## Respiration
- Our aerobic capacity will diminish because less oxygen will be available to reach the blood.

## Excretory
- Our kidneys will become less efficient because we'll lose fluid capacity.
- We may experience incontinence because our bladder will lose its ability to hold fluid. This is especially true for people over 60 (19 percent of women and 8 percent of men).

## Eating
- Because we'll have less gastric juices to process what we eat, with advancing age our ability to digest protein, iron, calcium, vitamin $B_{12}$, and folic acid will become impaired (by about 25 percent by age 60).
- We will not be able to maintain adequate levels of vitamins A and E, so to make up for this we might expect to take more vitamin supplements.

## Autonomic Nervous System

◆ Besides having less insulation, we may avoid recreational and other pleasurable activities because our ability to detect lower body temperature and our capacity to raise our body temperature when needed will diminish.

◆ We'll be more prone to get less rest when sleeping because during sleep our ability to breathe as freely as we once did will worsen. This is called *sleep apnea.*

◆ After age 60, *rapid eye movement* sleep (REM), the stage of sleep when most dreams occur, will get shorter. Because REM sleep assists in the transfer and storage of short-term memories into long-term memories, shorter REM sleep can mean an increase in intellectual decline.

## Reproductive

◆ Hormonal changes of menopause may make it more difficult for women to enjoy sexual activity due to changes in vaginal dryness, narrowness, and decreased vaginal length. Women's attitudes and values, though, play a bigger role in sexual gratification than do hormonal changes.

◆ Men may have more difficulty urinating because the prostate enlarges with age. It may also be more difficult for men to be sexually aroused or to maintain an erection because the sexual response cycle of men slows with age.

## Central Nervous System

◆ Acetylcholine, the brain chemical believed to be critical in memory, naturally declines.

◆ Our ability to concentrate, focus, and sustain our attention will decline because the level of *dopamine,* another important brain chemical, will also decline.

## Vision

◆ We will have a greater need for reading glasses because our ability to see objects nearer to us will decline. This is known as *presbyopia.*

◆ Our ability to operate a car at night will diminish because our night vision and ability to adapt to the dark will decline with age.

## Hearing

- ◆ We'll lose some of our ability to hear human voices clearly because our sensitivity to higher tones (especially for men) diminishes with age.

## Taste

- ◆ We may enjoy foods less or may use more salt or sugar to enhance their taste because with advancing age we'll have more difficulty detecting the subtleties of foods.

## Thinking Abilities

- ◆ We'll process information more slowly and be less mentally quick. What this means is that the speed and accuracy of our thinking and perceptions will be slower.
- ◆ We'll have more trouble coordinating our motor skills with what we see and hear, so we will be less quick on our feet.
- ◆ As we advance into old age, we will have more trouble integrating or sorting out irrelevant information, so we may get more easily distracted, we may get more easily confused by complex information, or we may quickly jump to erroneous conclusions.
- ◆ And finally, what's called *working memory* will naturally decline—that is, our ability to concentrate and attend to what we hear and see will decrease, so with advancing age our capacity to juggle facts in our head will naturally diminish. It is these deficits in working memory that best explain those "senior moments."

It's important to appreciate that all these predictable changes in later life have profound psychological and emotional implications, as well. For example, as we lose a sense of our own youth and vigor, we may become more fearful of losing our balance or of falling, and to compensate, we might try to restrict our activities. We may walk more cautiously or may move with less confidence. This can have an unintended consequence—when we start to cut ourselves off from the things that provide us pleasure we may unwittingly be setting ourselves up for depression. Increasingly aware that we are losing our endurance or that our bladders may sometimes fail us can be nagging reminders of our own mortality, and this raises the potential for arousing anxiety or even panic. Deficits in our cognitive abilities can lead to self-doubt and self-conscious performance anxiety. These are some of the challenges we'll face in coping with advancing age.

Here's the good news, though. Our vocabulary, our ability to do arithmetic, our ability to apply useful information accumulated over the years, and our comprehension of what we read or hear will all remain quite stable. In fact, these components of verbal intelligence can be expected to remain stable until at least age 80! And our vocabulary will maintain its stability to age 90!

Because we can expect decline in our thinking capacities, does that imply that common forgetfulness is a sign of impending Alzheimer's? Definitely not! How can we alert ourselves to what may be Alzheimer's? How is Alzheimer's different from normal aging? This is the business of the next few chapters.

As much as we might hope for something different, we begin to live life on life's terms when we accept the inevitability of change. It is then that we can become truly happy. By doing so, we can let go of expectation, go with the flow, and begin to embrace what is truly before us. This is one of those homework assignments we have in life, and it is especially true for those with Alzheimer's and for those who provide care to them.

# 3

# Alzheimer's Is a Type of Dementia

"Every life has a measure of sorrow.
Sometimes it is this that awakens us."

Alzheimer's is just one of many different types of dementia. Dementia is a category of illnesses characterized by problems in thinking, learning, memory, language, perception, and judgment. Of all the dementias, Alzheimer's is the most common. Out of 100 people who are diagnosed with dementia, roughly 55 of them will have Alzheimer's. The diagnosis of Alzheimer's dementia is called a *diagnosis of exclusion*—that is, it is a diagnosis that is made when all other types of dementia and other illnesses have first been ruled out. Shown in table 3a is a list of the most common types of dementia and their frequency of occurrence.[1]

The second most common type of dementia is called *vascular dementia* and is usually caused by a *stroke,* a vascular blockage in the brain. In addition to deficits in thinking, people who have had strokes often have problems with walking or with paralysis of their limbs, usually occurring on the opposite side of the body from where the brain blockage has occurred. For example, when a stroke occurs in the left half of the brain, speech and language

**Table 3a.** Frequency of the Various Types of Dementia

| Type of Dementia | Percentage of All Dementias |
|---|---|
| Alzheimer's dementia | 55% |
| Vascular dementia (often called a "stroke") | 20% |
| Frontotemporal dementia (e.g., Pick's disease) | 10% |
| Lewy body dementia (e.g., Parkinson's disease) | 10% |
| Dementia due to . . . | |
| Normal pressure hydrocephalus | 5% |
| HIV | 1% |
| Head trauma | 1% |
| Huntington's disease | 1% |
| Creutzfeldt-Jakob's disease | 1% |
| Persistent substance abuse | 1% |
| Other general medical conditions | 1% |

(located in the left half of the brain) might be affected while the right half of the body may show signs of paralysis. Strokes can be very serious and cause permanent impairment, but many times they can be effectively treated with medicines and physical rehabilitation. The initial thinking was that vascular dementia and Alzheimer's developed and progressed along two separate and distinct pathways. Newer research, however, indicates that Alzheimer's is also triggered by vascular risk factors.[2]

*Frontotemporal* dementia (of which Pick's disease is a type) is characterized by disturbances in personality and interpersonal relationships, degeneration in language abilities, or changes in movement and muscle function. Dementia can also be caused by *Parkinson's disease,* a movement disorder characterized by muscle rigidity, slowing of movement, and problems walking. Impairments in thinking characteristic of dementia will occur in the later stage of Parkinson's. Dementia caused by *normal pressure hydrocephalus* is a treatable condition that occurs when there is a buildup of fluid in the brain. By some estimates, this type of dementia accounts for 5 percent of all dementia cases.[3] When fluid pressure builds in the brain, problems with memory, walking and standing, and urinary (and sometimes bowel) incontinence can occur. Among other causes, dementia can also be brought about by head injuries or by the long-standing and persistent abuse of alcohol. Later in their lives, boxers will often suffer from dementia due blows to their head—when this occurs it's called *dementia pugilistica,* or being "punch drunk." When all the medical causes are tallied, there are more than 30 different types of dementia, and about 10–15 percent of people who have dementia have what's called a *mixed dementia*—that is, more than one type at the same time. People who have a degenerative dementia (like Alzheimer's, Parkinson's, or frontotemporal dementia) may also have what are called *Lewy bodies.* By some physicians' way of thinking, Lewy body dementia (LBD) may be present in 10 percent of otherwise identified cases of dementia. Lewy body dementia involves cognitive impairment, but its course can fluctuate significantly throughout the day. The memory of the person with LBD is usually quite good, but periods of confusion, movement, and motor problems, bent posture, visual-spatial difficulties, and visual hallucinations punctuate the illness. LBD patients who are given antipsychotic medications are three to four times more likely, though, to develop severe side effects. All of the other types of dementia put together, however, are less common than Alzheimer's.

## Cognitive Signs and Symptoms of Alzheimer's Dementia

So far, we have looked at some of the physical evidence that marks Alzheimer's disease. But as I also have discussed, Alzheimer's is not only a physical illness, it is a mental illness as well. Everyday difficulties in thinking and emotion are considered *psychiatric disorders* when certain signs and symptoms become problematic enough to impair social or occupational functioning. The American Psychiatric Association has developed standards for identifying exactly what should be considered psychiatric diagnoses and the symptoms comprising them. What follows is a list of the signs and symptoms necessary to qualify for a psychiatric diagnosis of Alzheimer's dementia:[4]

1. There must be significant memory problems—as evidenced by deficits in immediate recall, short-term memory, or long-term memory.
2. There must be significant thinking problems—as evidenced by problems in at least one of the following four areas of functioning:
   ◆ *Aphasia*—problems with expressing or comprehending language;
   ◆ *Agnosia*—problems identifying familiar things by sight, smell, sound, or touch;
   ◆ *Apraxia*—poor coordination, abnormal reflexes or gait, muscle weakness, stiffness, or paralysis; and
   ◆ *Problems in executive functioning*—deficits in higher-order thinking, such as planning, organizing, or making sound judgments.

3. The memory and thinking problems must be severe enough to cause significant decline in the quality of relationships with others or in a person's work performance.
4. The symptoms must have come on gradually (contrasted with a stroke, for example, where the problems come on all at once).
5. The problems must not be caused by another medical condition (like a brain tumor or persistent alcohol abuse) or by delirium (a disturbance in consciousness to be explained in more detail in chapter 5) or by another psychiatric disorder (like schizophrenia or major depression).

In the early stages of Alzheimer's, memory problems are limited to difficulties recalling recently learned material. It's a person's short-term memory that initially is most profoundly affected by Alzheimer's. For example, many of my Alzheimer's patients have difficulty remembering the last time a relative had visited them or when they last took their medications. One of my highly intelligent elderly patients, a longtime sports nut, told me that he watched the sporting news every day. As it turned out, I interviewed him on the morning of baseball legend Ted Williams's death. When I asked him what he had just seen on that morning's news, he replied, "This morning a guy died, a sports figure. He was ancient. I forgot his name." As the disease progresses, long-term memory becomes affected. When asked to tell me about her children, one of my patients replied, "I think my two children are named after my brother." Actually, this patient had a third child as well, a daughter. Another one of my patients was quite articulate, but when asked if she had any children (which she did not), she offered the names of her two cats. When recall memory is poor, sometimes prompting the person can help—that is, the person with Alzheimer's may be able to recall what they want to say when given a clue. For example, although unable to recall the name of her power of attorney, a patient of mine was able to recognize it among a list of other names.

About one-third of Alzheimer's sufferers are completely unaware they have memory problems. This can be due to emotional denial or because of an impairment stemming directly from the disease. About one-third are keenly aware they have the disease, and about one-third have partial awareness. In order to compensate for what they cannot recall or to deliberately mask their memory problems from others, people with Alzheimer's will often concoct responses that may have just enough truth to them to make some sense. This is called confabulation. For example, when asked why she was in my office for a competency evaluation, one of my elderly patients sweetly stated,

"I got a notice, dear." When asked to elaborate what notice she had received, she assertively replied, "It was time to get a checkup." Despite having been given prompts to jar her memory for what her son had told her right before the interview, this patient was not able to recall why she was being evaluated. To compensate, she nonetheless attempted to formulate a response that seemed to make sense to her. When a person knows her memory is failing, she may use others as external memory aids to compensate. For example, when asked why she was there in my office to see me for a competency evaluation, another one of my patients stated without hesitating, "If Vivian [her caseworker who was seated next to her] says I should be here, then I should."

In order to get a better sense of the degree to which people with Alzheimer's experience memory problems, try a brief mental test by looking at the lists shown in figure 3a.[5] First, cover columns 2 and 3 with a sheet of paper. Then read each item in the first column aloud, and commit it to memory. Now, cover columns 1 and 3 and do the same for the word set in column 2. Covering columns 1 and 2, then read column 3 aloud and commit it to memory. In five minutes and without looking, try to recall as many of the words from the lists as you can. If you score 8 or more consider yourself "Very Sharp." If you score 3–7 consider yourself "Normal." But if you score 2 or less, it's an indication of early Alzheimer's.[6] The word indication is important here; it implies that memory problems alone are not sufficient to qualify for a diagnosis of Alzheimer's. You must exhibit at least one of the other symptoms listed in the criteria I provided above, about which I will talk more about next. Besides Alzheimer's, many other things could account for a low score on this test.

**Figure 3a.** A Quick Memory Test for Alzheimer's

| | | |
|---|---|---|
| leg | cup | stamp |
| cheese | flower | leg |
| tent | forest | flower |
| motor | leg | cheese |
| flower | cheese | king |
| stamp | tent | menu |
| cup | stamp | motor |
| king | king | cup |
| forest | menu | tent |
| menu | motor | forest |

Adapted from Snowdon (2001).

Aphasia is one of the most common problems in Alzheimer's and is the label used to describe difficulties in the comprehension or expression of language. One of my well-read Alzheimer's patients once told me, "My reading is not too good . . . my eyes get in the way." Another patient who had been employed as a roofer told me, "I feel down and blue. I can't get the pen going." He went on to describe his occupation by stating, "I done the correction. I put bad wood back into it." When asked to spell the word "WORLD," another one of my well-educated patients replied, "W-O-R-L-V." A patient of mine recently told me that he eats [raisin] bran flakes in the morning "with the black things in it." One of my dearest Alzheimer's patients, who had visual hallucinations of passenger airplanes stuck in the tree outside her window, could never remember the word "psychologist," and when asked one day if she remembered who I was, blurted out, "You're 'The Nutcracker'!" We laughed and laughed, and she felt good that she had a new title she could use for me. These are all examples of language impairments.

It's important to note here that aphasia comes in two forms: *expressive aphasia* and *receptive aphasia.* Just because people with Alzheimer's may not be able to express themselves as articulately as they once could does not necessarily mean that they cannot understand what you tell them. These are separate problems that may or may not be manifest at the same time and would depend on how the disease has developed. More formal psychological testing might reveal that the Alzheimer's patient may be able to name in 60 seconds only four or five items he might find in a grocery store but would know what the words meant when they were used by others. One of my elderly patients described aphasia quite well when he said, "I know what I want to say but I can't put it into words. There is something there I just can't get a hold of. You know I know!"

*Agnosia* (problems in identifying familiar things by sight, sound, smell, or touch) is a symptom most frequently manifest in the later stages of Alzheimer's. This is because Alzheimer's is a disease that spreads toward the back of the brain, and sensory and motor functions located toward the top and back of the brain are affected only later in the disease. A common manifestation of agnosia occurs when a person is unable to recognize nursing staff or even family members. In a particularly severe case, a 91-year-old patient of mine could identify a pencil when held in front of him but identified my eyeglasses as "sick babies." Mistakes like this might also be the result of aphasia as well as agnosia. Another patient of mine was unable to recognize me despite having seen me once a week for many months.

Symptoms of *apraxia* are present when the body loses its ability to carry out small motor tasks. One type of apraxia occurs when the task to be performed is requested by someone else. For example, raising one of her arms above her head or tapping on the table might be something a person with Alzheimer's can do perfectly well if she were removing her clothing or knocking on a door, but when asked directly to do so out of context, she may be unable to carry out the request. This problem is called *ideomotor apraxia* and occurs because the language and motor centers of the brain are not communicating well enough with each other. Another type of apraxia, called *ideational apraxia,* occurs when a short sequence of movements cannot be performed. Driving an automobile, getting dressed, and preparing or eating a meal all require the ability to perform many small tasks in sequence. Some Alzheimer's patients are unable to copy simple drawings or to even sign their own names without distorting or rotating them. This type of apraxia occurs because the spatial and motor areas of the brain aren't in sync. About half of those with mild Alzheimer's might be considered capable of driving safely. After one to two years, few, if any, would.

*Executive functioning impairments* or problems in higher-order thinking and judgment can also be key symptoms of the illness. One of my patients had flooded her apartment with water from a running toilet that was clogged but neglected. She never thought to attend to the problem. Many of my patients have been deceived or unscrupulously swindled by others. Among other reasons, this occurs when there are executive functioning impairments. Like all deficits in Alzheimer's, the severity of executive functioning deficits will vary among those with the illness.

Michael was one of my patients who could not sufficiently manage his money on his own. Because of this, the court had decided to grant financial guardianship to his son. Michael knew the purpose and method of writing checks to his corner grocer, however, and as a result, he was granted the liberty to do so by the court. Another one of my patients was quite sharp and could easily solve simple arithmetic problems. She was given a financial guardian, though, because she was judged incompetent to manage her $50 million portfolio.

As a way of measuring patients' level of executive functioning, clinicians will often ask them to explain various proverbs. They might ask the person to explain the meaning of the phrase "When the cat's away the mice will play." One of my Alzheimer's patients responded to this by stating, "Why, they're not home!" This is due to an impairment in abstract thinking—an executive functioning deficit. Another proverb I've given Alzheimer's patients to explain is "Even monkeys fall out of trees." One of my colleagues told me that one of his patients had replied to this proverb by saying, "That's because the odd ones don't." In very severe cases, a person with Alzheimer's will not be able to identify the opposite of "up" or "large" or describe how an apple and an orange are alike.

Although I have distinguished between memory problems, aphasia, agnosia, apraxia, and executive functioning, these intellectual functions may not be independent of one another but in fact may overlap, sometimes making it difficult to distinguish one from another. To take an example, say someone suffering from Alzheimer's is unable to explain to you why she is not closing the door after she enters the house as she has promised you she would do. Several explanations are possible: (1) she might be forgetting to do it, (2) she might not know how to put her explanation into words, (3) she might not realize that closing the door is useful for safety reasons and to save energy and expense, or (4) she might not be able to translate her thought, "I need to close the door," into action. Thinking deficits like these can be more finely distinguished from one another by a clinician trained in working with the elderly.

## Common Emotional and Behavioral Problems in Alzheimer's

Alzheimer's can be better understood by categorizing its symptoms into three domains: cognitive deficits, functional impairments, and emotional and behavioral problems. It is estimated that 80 percent of people with Alzheimer's in the middle of its course have some type of emotional or behavioral symptoms such as irritability, apathy, depression, or psychotic symptoms. In an initial interview, a daughter of one of my patients once told me, "If it wasn't for the wandering, I think we could handle things at home with Mom." Although the diagnosis of Alzheimer's is based primarily on deficits in memory and thinking, what causes the most stress for family members and other caregivers are the afflicted person's unpredictable actions and inconsolable feelings.[7] These behaviors and emotional disturbances invariably have profound effects on the Alzheimer's sufferer and are one of the most commonly observed indications of the disease. Some of the most common emotional disturbances are apathy and lethargy, delusions, irritability and agitation, excessive worry, sleep disturbances, and depression.[8] See appendix D, table 1 for a more thorough list of emotional disturbances in dementia and their frequency of occurrence.

Because people with Alzheimer's are less able to regulate their own emotions, internal reactions like these cannot be effectively contained. When

**Figure 3b.** Behavior Problems Commonly Seen in Alzheimer's Disease

◆ Wandering and restlessness

◆ Repeatedly asking questions

◆ Unusual suspiciousness

◆ Frequently losing or misplacing things

◆ Decreased initiation; starting but not finishing things

◆ Talking little or not at all; social withdrawal

◆ Seeing or hearing things that aren't there

◆ Excessive irritation, anger, argumentativeness, or aggressiveness

◆ Decreased ability to manage relationships

◆ Behavioral disinhibition (e.g., shoplifting, inappropriate sexual advances, public urination)

◆ Hiding things

◆ Sleep disturbances

◆ Worry or anxiety

◆ Overdependency, clinging behavior, excessive demands

◆ Excessive euphoria or giddiness

◆ Misinterpreting sights or sounds

◆ Hyperactivity, excessive fretfulness

◆ Decreased ability with tasks such as grooming, dressing, toileting, eating, bathing, or walking

◆ Decreased ability with tasks such as shopping, traveling, paying bills, preparing meals, managing one's own health, insuring one's own safety, or communicating effectively

this happens, these internal reactions wind up getting acted out in odd and potentially disruptive behavior. When feelings and disturbing thoughts are not discussed, processed, and worked through, they will likely be acted out in action or be manifest in a greater frequency of health complaints. Contained in figure 3b are some of the most common behavioral problems that are found with Alzheimer's.[9]

My wife, Lori, had spent many years as a nurse working with people with Alzheimer's, and she recounted to me with fondness a story about one of her most cherished clients. In doing so, she provides us with a vivid illustration of how Alzheimer's can paradoxically be so perplexing and yet, at the same time, so understandable.

> Her memory and understanding of her current life were gone, but when I arrived at her home, Ms. Charlotte would cup my face with her hands, and with a beautiful smile and shining eyes would softly and slowly say, "Remember . . . you've *got* to have *fun!*" as if it were the secret of life. She would say this from the depth of her spirit, and her eyes would speak

her truth. Then she would ask me to dance . . . and off we would glide through the house. One day, in her wanderings, she walked into her bedroom, and I heard a clang, like something had fallen. I walked in to see her holding around her head the long lace window curtain like a wedding veil with a long train. Veil in hand, she began to walk the long hallway, curtain rod clanging behind her. At first I thought, "I must reorient her to reality . . . take the curtain away from her before she trips on it and hurts herself." Then I watched her as she approached the mirror, saying with joy, "Aren't I delightful!" I couldn't help but say, "Yes, you really are!" I then just slid the curtain rod out of the curtains and allowed her to parade through her home like a glorious bride.[10]

Life is bittersweet. What makes it so is that its splendor is always cast in the foreground of its disappointments. We can never avoid life's misfortune, but when we accept this incontrovertible idea we become awake to how precious all the glorious moments of our life can become.

# 4

# Evidence of Alzheimer's

"On a withered tree, a flower blooms."[1]

How can you definitely identify that it's Alzheimer's? The only way to diagnose Alzheimer's disease with absolute certainty is for a brain surgeon to conduct a biopsy or for a pathologist to conduct an autopsy after the person's death. Therefore, when someone is diagnosed with Alzheimer's the diagnosis is appropriately indicated in a tentative manner as *possible Alzheimer's* or *probable Alzheimer's*. To diagnose the possible or probable presence of Alzheimer's, clinicians can infer the presence of the disease only after they've done the following:

1. Collected historical and behavioral information from the person,
2. Completed a thorough physical examination,
3. Collected a thorough history from the person's family, and
4. Ruled out other medical or psychiatric causes that might explain the symptoms just as well.

To rule out other causes for the symptoms they might be observing, physicians might conduct blood tests or they might order a CT-scan or magnetic resonance image (MRI). Blood tests may show uncommonly low levels of folic acid (a B-complex vitamin) or low levels of vitamin $B_{12}$ (a vitamin important in memory) or high levels of homocysteine (an essential amino acid). Abnormal blood levels such as these are often found in people with Alzheimer's.[2] Because low folic acid and vitamin $B_{12}$ levels are also commonly found in chronic alcoholics, the physician must begin a process to narrow down all the possible medical conditions that could explain what is being observed. Figure 4a presents a list of other diseases that can mimic many of the symptoms of Alzheimer's.[3]

As you can see, the same symptoms that look like Alzheimer's could also be caused by cardiovascular problems, metabolic problems, an infection, a tumor, and so on. Therefore, the clinician would need to rule these out before concluding that Alzheimer's is the most likely cause.

## Microscopic Evidence of Alzheimer's

Microscopic evidence, found by a surgeon or pathologist, is the most conclusive evidence of Alzheimer's. The brain weighs about 3 pounds; it has about 100 billion nerve cells; and it has about 100 trillion points of connection between those cells. But knowing what to look for, a pathologist might observe under a microscope or from an imaging scan evidence of the following:[4]

◆ *Amyloid plaques* (sometimes called *senile plaques*)—these occur when pockets or clusters of the protein *beta-amyloid* are surrounded by dead neurons. A picture of an amyloid plaque is shown in figure 4b.

◆ *Neurofibrillary tangles*—these are present when pairs of neurons become twirled around one another and look like short jump ropes that are twisted together. Mutations in a protein, called *tau,* are believed to affect the "skeletal" structure of neurons that lead them to tangle around one another, and I will discuss more about this later on in this chapter. These neurofibrillary tangles are shown in figure 4c.

◆ *Granulovacuolar degeneration of neurons*—this occurs when pockets or vacuoles within the cells of the brain fill with fluid and granular substances.

◆ *Neuronal loss*—this occurs when neurons lose their mass. There may also be a loss in the total number of neurons that are present.

◆ *Synaptic loss*—losses may occur in the space or gap between nerves (called the *synapse*) where chemicals (called *neurotransmitters*) are released and reabsorbed. These neurotransmitters travel from one nerve to another and allow the nerves to communicate with one another.

**Figure 4a.** Some Common Medical Conditions Whose Symptoms Can Be Similar to Alzheimer's

**Psychiatric disorders**
◆ Dementia syndrome of depression

**Endocrine and metabolic disorders**
◆ Vitamin deficiency
◆ Hypothyroidism or hyperthyroidism
◆ Cushing's disease
◆ Kidney or liver failure

**Infection**
◆ Syphilis
◆ AIDS

**Vascular disease**
◆ Heart attack
◆ Stroke

**Brain tumor**

**Head trauma**

**Degenerative disorders**
◆ Huntington's disease
◆ Parkinson's disease
◆ Frontotemporal dementia

**Toxic drug levels**
◆ Alcohol
◆ Carbon monoxide
◆ Medication interactions
◆ Excessive medications

**Other conditions**
◆ Epilepsy
◆ Multiple sclerosis
◆ Normal pressure hydrocephalus

**Figure 4b.** A Close-Up View of an Amyloid Plaque (Dark Center) with Surrounding Neural Degeneration

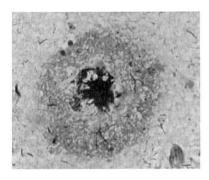

*Photo courtesy of Dennis J. Selkoe, M.D., Brigham and Women's Hospital, Boston.*

The medical and scientific communities have developed some very powerful imaging tools to look for and identify Alzheimer's. Here's a very brief primer on what's available. The *computed (axial) tomography,* or CT, scan was the first of these. Like an X-ray, a CT scan uses radiation to make image slices of the brain. It can identify gross changes in overall brain loss but is really better for imaging bones than it is brain matter. It is, however, the least expensive of the imaging methods at about $1,200 a scan.

**Figure 4c.** An Electron Microscopic View of Neurofibrillary Tangles

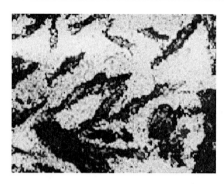

*Photo courtesy of R. D. Terry, University of California, San Diego.*

*Magnetic resonance imaging* (MRI) does not use radiation but changes in magnetic charge to detect brain loss. MRIs produce a clearer image and are better in detecting detail in soft fluid and soft tissue but cannot be used when pacemakers or metal plates or clips are present. An MRI costs about $2,000. At about the same price, the clinician can also ask for a functional MRI. This imaging tool provides structural information like an MRI but also provides detailed information about blood flow.

A much more powerful imaging method to detect Alzheimer's is *positron emission tomography* (PET). PET scans are much more expensive (ranging from $3,000 to $6,000) and use radiation like a CT scan but provide a direct measure of biological activity of very high clarity and resolution. A newer addition to the tomography imaging family but less frequently available is the *single photon emission computed tomography* (SPECT). A SPECT scan can recognize very small changes in brain activity with high resolution at a cost of about $1,000. It also uses radiation. Shown in figure 4d is a photo of a SPECT scan of an Alzheimer's patient.

## Evidence of Abnormal Neurotransmitter Levels

There are nearly 45 different neurotransmitters in the brain, but four of them are usually considered to be the most important—*acetylcholine, serotonin, norepinephrine,* and *dopamine.* Each of them has a specific function that is described in figure 4e, and when Alzheimer's is present there can be evidence of the following changes in neurotransmitter levels:

**Figure 4d.** SPECT Scan of an Alzheimer's Patient

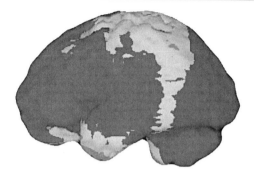

Lighter areas on the scan indicate diseased tissue.

*Much appreciation is offered to Brain Matters, Inc., 201 University Blvd., Suite 200, Denver, CO 80206, (877) 570-2650, for the courtesy of letting me use some of their scans and educational material.*

**Figure 4e.** Functions of Four of the Most Important Neurotransmitters

*Acetylcholine*—vital to learning and memory
*Serotonin*—helps to control mood, appetite, sleep, and aggression
*Norepinephrine*—controls alertness, wakefulness, and adrenaline
*Dopamine*—controls movement and attention

◆ Decreased *acetylcholine* levels—the primary brain chemical involved in learning and memory;

◆ Increased *acetylcholinesterase* levels—the chemical that breaks down acetylcholine into its component parts so it can be reused;

◆ Decreased *choline acetyltransferase* levels—the chemical that puts the parts of acetylcholine back together; and

◆ Decreased *norepinephrine* levels—the brain chemical that controls alertness and wakefulness.[5]

## Evidence That Can Be Seen with the Naked Eye

Although similar but less prominent changes can be found in the normal elderly person, gross changes in the size and shape of the brain can be found in people with Alzheimer's. Changes such as these are shown in figure 4f.

When these changes are pronounced they are indicative of Alzheimer's and include the following:

**Figure 4f.** Gross Changes in the Alzheimer's Brain (*left*) and the Normal Brain (*right*)

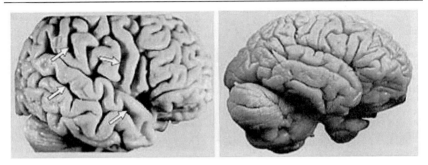

Note the large spaces (indicated by the white arrows) in the Alzheimer's brain where the brain has lost mass due to neural degeneration.

*Photo of the Alzheimer's brain courtesy of Anthony D'Agostino, M.D. Photo of the normal brain copyright © Dan McCoy/Rainbow.*

- *Diffuse atrophy*—the brain gets smaller and loses weight;
- *Flattened cortical sulci*—the natural brain separations become wider; and
- *Enlarged cerebral ventricles*—the natural fluid pockets in the brain get larger.

## Abnormal Genes

As I discussed earlier, plaques and tangles are the microscopic evidence of Alzheimer's. Much of what comprises plaques is beta-amyloid, which is believed to be the cause of the neural degeneration. Neurofibrillary tangles are believed to be caused by mutations in a chemical called tau, which can be measured in spinal fluid. In this section, I would like to take a closer look at beta-amyloid, tau, and what research on genetics and molecular biology has taught us about possible causes of Alzheimer's.

To begin this excursion into the microscopic world of Alzheimer's, let's first get some of the terms straight. A pictorial summary of what follows is contained in figure 4g.

In a nutshell, every cell in the body contains *DNA*—the code that identifies human (and most other) life. DNA combines to form *genes,* which act like instructions that are used to construct different molecules. A gene is about 100 to 2 million times the size of DNA. Scientists working for the Human Genome

**Figure 4g.** The Basics of Molecular Biology

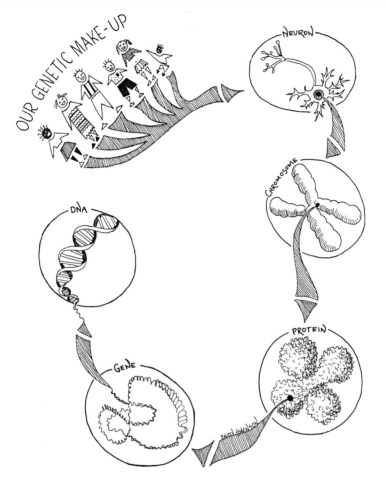

*Image courtesy of Betty Swenson.*

Project estimate that there are about 25,000 different genes that make up a human being. Genes combine to form *amino acids,* and if you link hundreds of amino acids together, you get an immense and complicated molecule called a *protein*—a molecule that organizes the structure, function, and regulation of processes within a cell. There are lots of different kinds of proteins, and one specific class of protein is called an *enzyme*—a protein that speeds up chemical reactions in the body. Take DNA and tightly wind it around another type of protein and you get a *chromosome.* Chromosomes are located in each cell nucleus, and there are 23 pairs of them in each normal cell.[6]

## Genetics and Familial Alzheimer's

As I talked about earlier, scientists looking into the causes and possible cures for Alzheimer's have based their research on two predominant lines of inquiry— (1) the amyloid hypothesis and (2) the cholinergic hypothesis—and recall that the amyloid hypothesis is based on the idea that neural degeneration occurs at brain sites where beta-amyloid has accumulated. Genetic and molecular biologists have discovered that beta-amyloid is a by-product of what's called the *amyloid precursor protein* (or APP, for short). When the processes producing APP and beta-amyloid are operating normally, these two proteins become essential in healthy cell functioning and growth.[7] When their operation goes awry, though, problems occur, so research scientists have been trying to figure out answers to two fundamental questions: (1) How does APP get formed? and (2) How does APP become transformed into toxic beta-amyloid?

In some people, deep inside the amyloid precursor protein a critical gene mutates. When this *APP-gene,* as it is referred to, is altered, a series of chemical events are set in motion that produce excessive amounts of beta-amyloid. This APP-gene is located on chromosome 21. As can be seen in figure 4h, mutations in the APP-gene trigger abnormal processing of the amyloid precursor protein, which, in turn, produces excessive beta-amyloid, which accumulates in amyloid plaques, and which eventually leads to cell degradation and cell death.

To be a little more specific, once gene mutation has contaminated the amyloid precursor protein, it is believed that two protein-cutting enzymes (referred to as beta-secretase and gamma-secretase) act as catalysts that sever the ends of the amyloid precursor protein, leaving a fragment of it in its wake. The fragment that is left behind is toxic beta-amyloid. Molecular and genetic scientists believe that if a drug could be created that could inhibit beta- and gamma-secretase enzymes, the unwanted production of beta-amyloid could be stopped, and I will talk a little more about that in chapter 12.[8]

Familial (early-onset) Alzheimer's is believed to arise from mutations in the APP-gene and two other genes that guide the construction of presenilin-1 (located on chromosome 14) and presenilin-2 (located on chromosome 1), both aptly named by their reference to the early or "pre-senile" onset of the illness.[9] Understanding these gene mutations, the production of beta-amyloid, and all the intervening steps may eventually provide physicians with an arsenal of medications to inhibit the progression of the disease. APP genetic mutations are much more common in familial Alzheimer's than in late-onset Alzheimer's, but

**Figure 4h.** How the Mutated APP-Gene Leads to the Death of a Cell

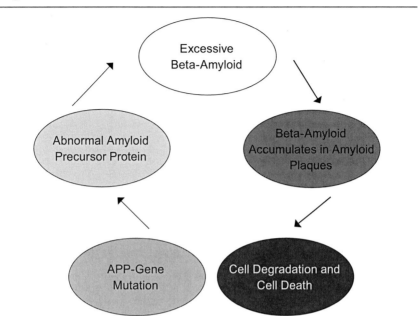

account for a small percentage of all familial Alzheimer's cases. Presenilin-1 and presenilin-2 mutations, however, are believed to account for a majority of the cases of familial Alzheimer's. A few mutations in APP and presenilin-2 have been identified, but over 130 different mutations in presenilin-1 have been found. Mutations in presenilin-1 are estimated to account for about 50 percent of the cases of familial Alzheimer's.[10]

Researchers have also found that mutations in chromosome 21 are present in people with Down's syndrome. Beta-amyloid levels have also been found to be higher in people with Down's syndrome. The similarities between Down's syndrome and Alzheimer's may help researchers better understand each of these disorders. There are gene mutations that put a person at greater risk for Alzheimer's, and there are genes that definitely lead to Alzheimer's. The genes that have been identified that definitely lead to the illness are called *deterministic genes* and are found in only a few hundred families worldwide and are much more likely to lead to early-onset Alzheimer's. Much of the research about these families is being conducted through the Dominantly Inherited Alzheimer's Network—a National Institute on Aging funded project through the Washington University School of Medicine.

## Genetics and Late-Onset Alzheimer's

From another branch of genetics research, it has been found that each person is born with two *apolipoprotein-E alleles* (two forms of a gene that are inherited from each parent). Researchers are especially interested in two of these alleles—ApoE-2 and ApoE-4. While the ApoE-2 allele may protect us from Alzheimer's, it's been found that the ApoE-4 allele (located on chromosome 19) may be responsible for an increase in beta-amyloid production. If a person inherits an ApoE-4 gene from each parent, his/her risk for Alzheimer's is the greatest. Just exactly how these gene variants affect Alzheimer's is not yet clear.[11] About 95 percent of all Alzheimer's cases are late-onset (after age 65), and although a range of percentages have been cited in the literature, about half of all Alzheimer's sufferers have the ApoE-4 allele. The problem is that so do about 25 percent of adults who do not have Alzheimer's. Research on ApoE continues, but at this time ApoE-4 is considered to be an unreliable clinical predictor of late-onset Alzheimer's.

The protein *tau* has also been associated with late-onset Alzheimer's. When nerve cells get twisted together in Alzheimer's, they are referred to as neurofibrillary tangles. Within a healthy nerve cell, the nutrients the cell needs to thrive travel down train-track-like cell parts called *microtubules.* Tau is a protein molecule that acts like railroad ties holding the microtubules together. It is believed that gene mutations on chromosome 17 lead to an altered form of tau, and when this happens the train-tracks get twisted, the nutrients don't get delivered effectively, and the cell begins to degrade. Researchers believe that neurodegenerative disorders like Alzheimer's can be better understood by using this frame of reference, and it is called the *tau hypothesis.* Scientists have discovered that high concentrations of aggregated tau can be found in the neurofibrillary tangles characteristic of Alzheimer's. Tau also aggregates in what are called *neuritic plaques,* which frequently surround amyloid clusters. Researchers believe that elevated tau levels could be an important biomarker for Alzheimer's, and tests have been devised to measure and compare tau levels from extracted cerebrospinal fluid.[12] Interestingly, ApoE-4 seems to bind to the beta-amyloid protein but not to the tau protein.

As I made reference to earlier, genes interact with environmental factors to produce Alzheimer's. For example, head injury is a risk factor for Alzheimer's, but it seems this may be the case only for people who carry ApoE-4. Floyd Patterson, the great heavyweight boxing champion, is a good example of this. Patterson died of Alzheimer's in 2006 at the age of 71. While it was widely speculated that his Alzheimer's was the consequence of head concussions, both of Patterson's parents died of the illness.

A gene that may have more influence than the ApoE-4—one that operates in the immune system and is referred to as the *receptor accessory protein* (RAP)—is believed to increase the risk for Alzheimer's. People who carry the RAP gene show higher rates of amyloid plaque buildup than those who don't. The RAP gene may also be associated with lower immune system functioning and greater temporal lobe atrophy.[13]

Finally, I would like to say a few words about the ethics of genetic testing. Late-onset Alzheimer's cannot be reliably predicted by a genetic test, but genetic testing could aid in the diagnosis of an individual who shows identifiable signs and symptoms of dementia. Many geneticists and medical ethicists take the position that genetic testing for Alzheimer's is not appropriate at this time.[14] The predominant opinion, however, is that genetic testing is more appropriate for genes associated with familial Alzheimer's than for late-onset Alzheimer's, but only for families where known mutations in Alzheimer's sufferers have been clearly identified.[15] A number of labs will conduct clinical genetic testing. There have been, however, a number of "direct-to-consumer" testing labs that have also emerged recently—in that they allow individuals to bypass those in the medical community—and caution is advised in considering them, because advice and counseling for interpreting test results are generally unavailable.[16]

A positive test result for Alzheimer's can be extremely anxiety-provoking, and a negative test result may falsely give the illusion of reassurance. Because the risks and benefits of genetic testing must be clearly understood before a person engages in genetic testing, accurate and supportive genetic counseling is strongly advised. Genetic testing for research purposes is currently available for many different genetic mutations, including APP, presenilin-1, presenilin-2, and ApoE-4.

## A Word about Aluminum

Over the years, a lot has been bandied about regarding the role that aluminum might play in Alzheimer's. Aluminum is a major component of the earth's crust. It's commonly found in drinking water, but it can also be found in processed cheese, baked goods, antacids, and antiperspirants. Curiously, aluminum is also a component of tetanus shots, some flu shots, and other vaccines, because aluminum helps them work better. About 20 years ago, though, some studies found higher rates of Alzheimer's in dialysis patients, which led to the suspicion that the aluminum from the needles might be involved. Newer research has also found trace amounts of aluminum in plaques and tangles, but it is generally not believed that aluminum is a major player in the progression of the disease. Recently, though, the role of copper, iron, and other metals in Alzheimer's has been examined, and more will be discussed about that in chapter 12. The FDA does not limit the quantity of aluminum in foods.

## Miriam

Miriam was a 52-year-old patient of my outpatient practice. Her deceased mother was diagnosed with Alzheimer's when she was 65, and Miriam was concerned she was developing some of the symptoms. Miriam was having a slightly difficult time remembering names and appointments as well as she usually had. She was very smart, and I told her that memory problems like hers were common in normal distraction, stress, and concentration problems inherent in depression, anxiety, and other mental states. She denied any significant mood problems, but because of her strong family history and to better identify and localize the problem, I administered a battery of psychological tests (I will talk more about these about in chapter 7). The tests showed that she was experiencing some very mild deficits in specific areas of cognitive functioning but that she did not qualify for a diagnosis of Alzheimer's, or mild cognitive impairment, for that matter. Needless to say, she was very relieved. I explained to her, though, that too much stress could reasonably account for the slight memory deficits she was having, and she confided to me that her work and family life over the last year had been very stressful. I recommended that she lower her stress and follow up with me if her symptoms persisted. I also suggested various prevention methods that I will discuss further in chapter 15 and told her that genetic testing was available for familial Alzheimer's but only if she first got some good genetic counseling.

Although there is no cure for Alzheimer's there can be healing in Alzheimer's. Healing is more than physical recovery from bodily symptoms. What I mean by this is that some people who *have* a disease do not necessarily *suffer* from it. While their bodies are being ravaged, their spiritual pathway to an open heart is clear. They feel connected, grateful—and they can even bloom—just like a flower can blossom on a dying tree. We are more than our bodies, and at any age, transformation and enlightenment are always possible.

# 5

# Distinguishing Between Delirium, Alzheimer's, and Other Dementias

> "The trouble is that you think you have time . . . [so] live every act as fully as if it were your last."

Sometimes, when I've misplaced my glasses or my pen I've thought that my wife or daughter must have taken them. It was never the case. I was just jumping to conclusions. When it comes to accusing your family of something, particularly if they are innocent, it's a good idea to first rule out all the other possible explanations. It's like that with diagnosing Alzheimer's, too. Here's a case in point: *Delirium* is a medical condition whose symptoms are like Alzheimer's, but they're not. When an elderly patient in the hospital experiences memory problems it may likely be due to delirium, but sometimes hospital staff jump to the conclusion that it's Alzheimer's. When this happens, a diagnosis of dementia is given prematurely when delirium could account for the symptoms just as well.

## What Is Delirium?

Alice was an 82-year-old dementia patient of mine who lived in a nursing home. For several weeks, I had been counseling her for depression when one day her condition changed dramatically. She didn't recognize me right away, as she always had, and it was difficult for her to focus her attention on what I was saying. That day, Alice didn't know what day it was—something unusual for her. Some of the staff felt she may have had a stroke or a *transient ischemic attack,* which is like a tiny, "silent" stroke. Others felt it was the early signs of Alzheimer's. These were reasonable guesses but ones that could only be made after ruling out delirium. Sometimes in the elderly, a dramatic change in thinking can occur when there is some kind of infection present. Because urinary tract infections are very common in nursing home residents, I took a wild guess and asked her if it burned when she urinated. She told me, "Why, yes it does!" So I informed her physician, a urine sample was taken, and a urinalysis was performed. When the test came back it was "positive," and she was placed on an antibiotic. Soon after that, her orientation and attention problems disappeared.

Delirium is not actually a disease but a *syndrome* (a cluster of commonly associated symptoms) that is caused by another, underlying medical problem. According to the American Psychiatric Association, to qualify for a diagnosis of delirium the following criteria must be met:[1]

1. There must be a disturbance of attention and awareness—that is, the person must be experiencing a reduced clarity of awareness of the things around him, along with a reduced ability to focus, sustain, or shift attention.
2. There must be a change in thinking ability—such as memory problems, disorientation, language disturbances, or disturbances in perception that are not better accounted for by a diagnosis of dementia.
3. The disturbance must develop over a short period of time—usually in hours to days, and with delirium it often fluctuates during the course of the day.
4. The disturbance must be caused by the physiological effect of a general medical condition, exposure to a toxin, side effect of a medication, or from substance abuse—not by dementia, schizophrenia, malingering, or another medical or psychiatric explanation.

As a consequence of a delirium, certain other characteristics are also commonly observed, such as drowsiness and personality changes such as apathy, irritability, bizarre behaviors, mood swings, disorientation, poor memory, distractibility, seeing or hearing things that aren't there, restlessness, suspiciousness, or paranoia.[2]

Delirium is quite common in hospital patients, especially when surgery is performed. In fact, about 10–25 percent of patients on a hospital medical-surgical unit experience delirium. As you might expect, it is even more common on intensive care and cardiac care units (in roughly 30 percent of the cases there). For patients who are getting hip surgeries, it is higher still (about 40–50 percent). For hospital patients age 65 and older, delirium is present in 30–40 percent of all cases. Delirium can be very dangerous. It has a three-month mortality rate as high as 25–35 percent and has a one-year mortality rate as high as 40–50 percent.[3]

Concussions, heart problems, infections, alcohol intoxication, malnutrition, thyroid problems, seizures, and other conditions all can cause delirium. Its symptoms can overlap with those of dementia, depression, mania, various psychotic conditions, and a number of other medical conditions. It is very common to find delirium in people who are prescribed a large number of medications—particularly when an older (tricyclic) antidepressant or earlier-developed antipsychotic is being prescribed. Vascular and cardiovascular problems, infections, medications, vitamin deficiencies, and many other factors can also cause delirium.[4] Curiously, most of these causes have their origin outside the brain, and as with any illness, a thorough physical examination is needed to determine what medical condition may be causing the problem.

I want to mention to you here about a particular kind of delirium that is often seen in people with Alzheimer's—it's called *sundowning*. Sundowning has been given its name because it usually occurs as late afternoon turns into early evening. This is when increased signs of confusion and agitation can emerge. As nighttime sets in, the person with Alzheimer's may begin wandering or becoming more disoriented, more restless, or more fearful. In some medical and academic circles, sundowning is considered a form of sleep disturbance—more specifically, a disruption in the sleep-wake cycle. Let me explain this further.

By way of background, every living thing on the planet—from flowers to insects to humans—has its own *circadian cycle* or rhythm that determines its pattern of activity and rest. For just about everything, it's about 24 hours. It turns out, though, that as we age, the time we spend awake increases, the time we are in rapid eye movement sleep (REM-sleep) decreases, and sometimes our circadian cycles get out of sync. This is what happens to many people with Alzheimer's.[5] The alternation of light and dark outside corresponds to our circadian cycles, and as it gets dark, people with Alzheimer's are less able to use their sight to identify familiar things and often lose track of the cues that help them orient themselves. This can spark fear, trigger intense feelings of isolation, and elicit what can become a terrifying experience. Research has found, though, that exposing Alzheimer's patients to bright light in the evening can lead to less evening agitation, better sleep, and increased daytime activity.[6] Here's an example.

As evening set in at the nursing home, Gene began calling out for help and getting more agitated. When the staff tried to calm him, Gene would typically get more combative, and as it got darker, he became more confused and tearful. His physician had prescribed an "as needed" order of Ativan (a fast-acting anti-anxiety medication), and when Gene became more anxious and disoriented the staff routinely administered an evening dose of it. As time went on, though, we found that something so simple as turning on his room lights earlier in the day often prevented Gene's sundowning symptoms from emerging.

### What's the Difference Between Alzheimer's and Delirium?

A couple of years ago, I found a green Ford Taurus I wanted to buy, and I told my wife, Lori, all about it. She liked everything about it—except that it was green. When she saw it she fell in love with it. "That's not green," she said. "That's turquoise! I love turquoise!" Small differences can be important. If you compare a list of causes of delirium and causes of dementia the two lists would have much in common, but some key differences would stand out.

With Alzheimer's, the symptoms appear gradually, often initially in very subtle ways; but when people have a delirium, the onset of symptoms is rapid—one day the symptoms are absent, the next they are prominent. Unlike Alzheimer's, symptoms of delirium will usually fluctuate throughout the day. Once the medical cause of the delirium is found and treated, its symptoms will disappear, usually in a few days. Attention deficits, always present in delirium, are usually absent in Alzheimer's.[7] In some research circles, it's believed that delirium takes on a form similar to Alzheimer's because both disorders involve decreased levels of acetylcholine (the neurotransmitter responsible for memory). More interested readers can take a look at appendix D, table 2, for a more thorough distinction between Alzheimer's and delirium.

## How Does Alzheimer's Differ from Other Dementias?

As we've discussed in the last chapter, there are many different of types or causes of dementia, including dementia caused by vascular problems, Parkinson's disease, persistent alcohol abuse, elevated fluid levels in the brain, and others. Just how the problems associated with each of these disorders develop and how they can be distinguished from Alzheimer's is what I will be briefly discussing here.

Vascular dementia is similar to Alzheimer's in the sense that memory, language, and motor functioning can be affected. When a person has a severe stroke, many of the symptoms are obvious and the physician can rule out Alzheimer's by observing the person's neurological symptom profile and through the use of high-tech imaging methods. When a stroke is mild, however, it may be very difficult to distinguish between the two disorders. How abruptly the symptoms begin is a key factor. With Alzheimer's the symptoms come on gradually; with vascular dementia, the symptom onset is abrupt. It's not foolproof, but a scoring system to help clinicians distinguish between the two disorders has been developed, and it is included in appendix D, figure 1.[8]

Alzheimer's is a disease of the *cerebral cortex,* the outer layer of the brain that controls higher-order mental functioning. Shown in figure 5a is a sketch of the brain featuring the cerebral cortex. The cerebral cortex is made up of four primary areas, or *lobes.* The *frontal lobe* controls speech, emotion, judgment, and insight. The *temporal lobe* controls memory and hearing. The *parietal lobe* controls basic movements, and the *occipital lobe* controls vision. Research has revealed that Alzheimer's begins in the hippocampus—a C-shaped brain part located in the temporal lobe and responsible for short-term memory and the conversion of short-term to long-term memory. More specifically, memory (and Alzheimer's) begins in the *entorhinal cortex*—a kind of "front door" or input to the hippocampus. As Alzheimer's progresses, it spreads through the hippocampus and then throughout other regions of the cerebral cortex. Because of this, it is called a *cortical dementia.* Other diseases, like Parkinson's disease and Huntington's disease, develop because of abnormalities in more inner recesses of the brain. Because of this fact, they are referred to as *subcortical dementias.*

Parkinson's disease is a movement disorder characterized by muscle rigidity, slowing of movement, and problems with walking. About 30 to 50 percent

**Figure 5a.** The Cerebral Cortex

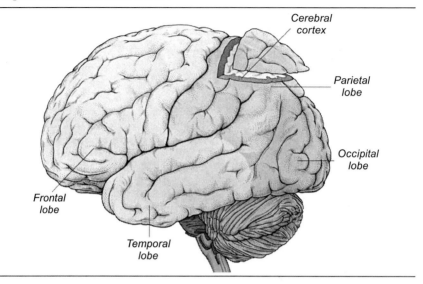

of the time, in the later stages of Parkinson's, symptoms of dementia emerge.[9] Dementia caused by Parkinson's is similar to Alzheimer's in that amyloid plaques and neurofibrillary tangles characteristic of Alzheimer's are often present in Parkinson's patients. But cortical dementias like Alzheimer's are character- ized by deficits in memory and language, whereas subcortical dementias, like Parkinson's, tend to show deficits in processing speed and executive function- ing.[10] For a more complete list of distinctions between cortical and subcortical dementia, see appendix D, table 3.

In Alzheimer's, the person is more often in good spirits and her speech and muscle coordination are usually functional until late in the disease, but she usually experiences significant word-finding difficulty. In subcortical dementias like Parkinson's, there is more often depression and muscular impairments in forming speech, but there is usually no difficulty in thinking or in finding words the person wants to say, especially early in the disease. These distinctions can be helpful to clinicians in determining which type of dementia is being observed and based on their conclusion, what other symp- toms might be expected.

I often find myself believing I can put things off—take care of them later—and this works for me some of the time. When it comes to saying and doing the things I need to do to love myself and others better, though, putting things off doesn't work so well. As I've gotten older, I like telling others how much I love them, holding more closely those unique and priceless moments—doing now what I formerly felt I could put off. This has brought me closer to the people I love and has helped me understand myself better. People with Alzheimer's and those who care for them each have things to share too. The beauty part of it is that each of them has a way of helping the other do this.

# 6

# Two Case Studies: Applying the Basics

"No matter how difficult the past, you can
always begin again today."

I've presented a great deal of information thus far, but as you continue to
review it, you will find it will sink in more and more. At this point, though,
I'd like to present a couple of examples to make the learnings come alive, so
let's take a short break and take a different look at some of the things we've
been discussing. Below I will be describing two case studies—one is about a
person who was admitted to the hospital and the other was someone I saw at
my outpatient practice. Your job is to try to figure out what issues are relevant
in determining whether the person has Alzheimer's disease, delirium, or what.
I want you to become a kind of detective and examine what the clues might
tell you. Take a look, and see what you can come up with.

## Mary in the Hospital

After she fell, Mary was admitted to the hospital for hip surgery. While she
was there, Mary began to show signs that she was having trouble with her
thinking. Her daughter was very concerned and asked someone from the

hospital to examine her. A psychologist came by and did an evaluation, and here's what he found:

- ◆ Mary was admitted for hip surgery following a fall she took in her home.
- ◆ Mary is 65 years old, college educated, African American, and a widow.
- ◆ She doesn't remember why she was admitted to the hospital.
- ◆ She's restless and suspicious of the nurses and other hospital staff.
- ◆ Mary lives alone, and her daughter lives out of state.
- ◆ She has a history of high cholesterol and hyperthyroidism.
- ◆ Mary's physical examination showed no remarkable neurological symptoms.
- ◆ She has no other family or social support in the area.
- ◆ Mary was to be discharged from the hospital to a nursing home for follow-up care.
- ◆ Mary insists on being discharged to her home.

Based on this information, what do you think was concluded from the evaluation? What should her daughter do about where her mother might live? What does the information say about Mary? Look over the clues. Which ones are potentially relevant? Is it dementia? Delirium? What? What questions would you want to ask the hospital doctors? Take a minute and think it over. Write down your thoughts. When you are done, take a look at what I have to say about it.

**Mary was admitted for hip surgery following a fall in her home**—Mary has fallen and as a consequence may have suffered a head trauma. Falls and other traumas, while dangerous in and of themselves, can also be indicative of a triggering stroke or transient ischemic attack. We've also learned that hip surgeries increase the likelihood of co-occurring delirium. Remember that delirium is medically caused and must be remedied before questions regarding other diagnoses like Alzheimer's can be resolved.

**Mary is 65 years old**—We've learned that Alzheimer's disease becomes more prevalent after age 65.

**She is college educated**—Higher education may mean less likelihood of showing signs of Alzheimer's, so if that's what's going on, it may also be more difficult for a clinician to pick up on the disease. Because she may be more articulate or witty, Mary may be better able to mask more serious signs of the illness.

**Mary is African American**—Recent research has shown that African Americans are slightly more likely to develop Alzheimer's than Euro-Americans. Also, because certain ethnic minorities have shorter life spans, Mary's functional age may be relatively older than her chronological age would imply.

**Mary is a widow**—As you might imagine and as we will learn later, this can imply bereavement or depressive issues, which can sometimes play out in the form of poor memory and concentration problems.

**She doesn't remember why she was admitted to the hospital**—This may be an understandable emotional reaction to the trauma of being hospitalized, it may be indicative of more serious short-term memory loss, or it may indicate trouble concentrating or focusing her attention. Memory problems alone may be indicative of delirium, dementia, depression, or some other condition.

**Mary is restless and suspicious of the nurses and hospital staff**—What we don't know about Mary is whether she had any personality problems prior to her fall, but restlessness and suspiciousness may be signals indicating more pervasive fears, paranoid reactions, or an inability to appropriately attend to, weigh, and evaluate outside information. All these are features of delirium, dementia, or other mental health conditions.

**She has a history of high cholesterol and hyperthyroidism**—These conditions raise the concern that cardiovascular abnormalities may be at play, thus implicating possible delirium- and dementia-related issues. Recent research has shown a link between the risk factors for Alzheimer's and vascular risk factors such as hypertension and high cholesterol.[1] Metabolic disturbances like hyperthyroidism also are possible causes of delirium and dementia-like symptoms.

**Mary's examination showed no remarkable neurological symptoms**—This would mean that Mary did not demonstrate any obvious signs of a stroke, Parkinson's, or Huntington's disease, for example. If any of these medical conditions was evident, though, it might also account for Mary's poor memory or decision making.

**Mary has no family or social support in the area**—This piece of information may be very important. How did this situation arise? Did Mary alienate others? Withdraw from others? This fact could raise concern about how Mary is handling interpersonal relationships, and this suggests the possibility of a mood disorder or other mental health condition. Recall that for many people with Alzheimer's, depression can be common in its early stages.

**Mary was to be discharged from the hospital to a nursing home for follow-up care, but she insists on being discharged to her home**—On the one hand, this is a natural response. Understandably, Mary wants to maintain her independence and autonomy. On the other hand, this fact raises concern about Mary's judgment. Good judgment is a higher-order executive function that is often clouded by Alzheimer's.

What did you come up with? Applying the right information can be tricky, but as you become more familiar with the factors involved, you will begin to get better at drawing the most appropriate and reasonable conclusions. In this case, the psychologist found memory and judgment problems and disorientation to time and to place that might be indicative of a dementia but also found that Mary had a greater level of difficulty focusing and sustaining her attention than would be expected in a dementia like Alzheimer's—something more often found in a delirium. As it turned out, Mary was experiencing a post-surgical delirium, and the hospital waited to see if it resolved on its own. In a couple of days, her symptoms remitted. Her better judgment returned, and she realized that she needed to be discharged to a nursing home for hip rehabilitation.

## Emmanuel: A More Complicated Case

Emmanuel was a 59-year-old, married, Caucasian male who was referred to my outpatient practice at the request of his psychiatrist. Over the last few years, he had been experiencing memory problems that had become so severe that he felt he needed to prematurely retire from a longtime professional career—one in which he had been quite competent and successful. He was currently depressed and had a decadelong history of *bipolar disorder* (what used to be called *manic depression*). He was taking eleven medications for a variety of conditions, including his bipolar disorder, hypertension, severe arthritis, stress incontinence, and high cholesterol. Emmanuel had been hospitalized some 20 years earlier with a closed-head injury and had since lost his memory for events leading up to the concussion. His psychiatrist felt he had a degenerative dementia (likely due to Alzheimer's) and had placed him on Aricept (an anti-dementia medication about which I will discuss more in chapter 12).

Over the last year, Emmanuel's symptoms had gotten steadily worse. These included substituting one alphabetic letter for another, calling things by their wrong names, problems paying bills, difficulty keeping score when playing cards, difficulty recalling his Social Security number, and difficulty remembering his grandchildren's names and ages. He had also been getting lost driving to familiar locations and was having trouble finding the right words to say exactly what he meant. About a year before I saw Emmanuel, his neurologist took a brain scan, which showed a small decrease in the size of his brain.

I assessed his mental status and administered a battery of cognitive tests (about which I will discuss more in chapter 7). The test results indicated that he qualified for a diagnosis of mild cognitive impairment. He had very mild signs of dementia, but he was able to compensate for them well enough to raise his scores up high enough to place him just outside the scores typical of diagnosed Alzheimer's patients. His test results also indicated, though, that his measured intelligence level was slightly lower than would be expected for someone with his scholastic record and professional work history.

What was going on with Emmanuel? Here was my take on it. I first wondered about a delirium from all the medications he was taking. I also wondered if the head trauma he experienced some 20 years earlier was having long-term effects on his memory and thinking. And then there was his psychiatric condition. As you will read more about in chapter 10, depression can look like dementia, and some of Emmanuel's symptoms, particularly his concentration and memory problems, might be explained by a depression. Finally, Emmanuel might also be experiencing the precursors of Alzheimer's. To say that Emmanuel has Alzheimer's, however, does not necessarily rule out the possibility that he may also be experiencing one or more of these other conditions, as well.

How to sort out these possibilities? What should be done next? Recall that Emmanuel's neurologist took an imaging scan of his brain the year prior to my evaluation of him. The next step for Emmanuel was to have his neurologist follow up with another brain scan to check for changes. His psychiatrist and family physician also were alerted, so that they could double-check his medications. If medication-induced effects were ruled out, it would be important to track key cognitive functions known to be sensitive to degenerative processes. Emmanuel's doctors decided to reduce the number of medications he was on, which helped reduce some of the symptoms he was experiencing, but it appeared that his cognitive impairments were most likely due to the aftermath of his head trauma or to Alzheimer's. As a result, supportive counseling was set up and a referral was made to a treatment program specializing in cognitive rehabilitation. Later on in the book, I will talk about more specific diagnostic follow-up tests that can further identify with greater certainty the diagnosis of Alzheimer's.

The nice thing about life is that, in a way, it starts out fresh every morning. Every day we get another chance to make it better, to make ourselves better, or perhaps make someone else better. This is our resplendent gift—that everything can begin anew. Despite the difficulties of yesterday, we have the chance to make at least a small piece of them right today. Those who provide care for Alzheimer's sufferers know this.

Part 2

# How to Evaluate for Alzheimer's

# 7

## This Person I Used to Know: Measuring the Status of Mental Functioning in Alzheimer's

"The mind contains all possibilities, but life is fleeting like a rainbow, a flash of lightning, a star at dawn."

### The First Step in a Thorough Assessment: Taking a Good History

Family members and friends are usually the first to see when something might be wrong. When someone has Alzheimer's, he is often unaware of it or he may deny that he is having thinking or memory problems. When this happens it's someone else who seeks out the help that's needed. What usually happens is a spouse or a son or daughter takes the person to see his family physician. When family members are not available or are not aware of the severity of the problem, friends or other people in the person's social support network must take this step. When no one else is available, a concerned neighbor might call *Adult Protective Services,* a county governmental service that safeguards the needs of the elderly in his community.

John, a patient I recently evaluated, was referred to me because his postal carrier continuously saw his house in disarray and observed John wearing the same clothes for days on end. At a loss for what else he could do, the mailman notified the regional office of the *Council on Aging,* which sent a nurse at no charge to John's home to conduct an evaluation. John's daughter was then contacted, and with results in hand, she scheduled an appointment with me to see her father.

Once a clinician gets involved, the first thing is to get an accurate history of the illness and its symptoms. Getting answers to certain key questions is vital in the clinician's initial assessment. The person being evaluated may be able to answer some of these questions on her own. For many of the questions, however, the person may need help from others. Here are some of the questions I usually ask in an initial screening interview:

1. Have you had any memory problems lately?
   - ◆ Have you misplaced frequently used or familiar objects?
   - ◆ Have you forgotten people's names you once knew well?
   - ◆ Have you gotten lost while traveling to a familiar location?
   - ◆ Are you concerned about the memory problems you've been having?
2. Have you had any trouble finding the right words to use or recalling the right names for things?
3. Have you had any trouble in any of the following areas?
   - ◆ Shopping?
   - ◆ Paying bills or handling finances?
   - ◆ Keeping appointments?
   - ◆ Preparing meals?
   - ◆ Managing your health?
   - ◆ Taking proper safety precautions?
   - ◆ Driving?
   - ◆ Communicating with others?
4. When were any changes first noticed?
5. Has someone else examined you or diagnosed the problem? Have any tests been done, like a CT scan, an MRI, or blood work?

6. Have any drugs been prescribed for your condition?
   - ◆ Can you name them?
   - ◆ Are you taking any other medications for any other medical condition?
   - ◆ Do you take them as prescribed?
7. Has the severity of the problem progressed gradually or in abrupt steps?
8. Have there been any serious falls or head injuries in the past?
9. Have you been diagnosed with a mental health or stress-related problem like depression or anxiety?
   - ◆ Has anyone else in your family been diagnosed with a stress-related problem or had a problem like this?
   - ◆ Have you experienced any mood swings or mood changes lately?
10. Has there been a time in your life when you were drinking much alcohol?

Many family physicians know their patients pretty well, and many of these diagnostic questions will have already been addressed. The physician will also routinely assess for neurological symptoms related to motor and sensory functioning, such as coordination problems, muscle weakness, dizziness, partial paralysis, vision disturbances, motor impairments, speech impairments, severe attention deficits, and so forth. Some of these symptoms may be relevant to a diagnosis of Alzheimer's. For example, in the early stages of Alzheimer's there is frequently an increased level of activity in deep tendon reflexes, reflexive reactions to painful or noxious stimuli, body rigidity or stooped posture, and in advanced stages, deficits in grasping or sucking ability. Specific results from this assessment can raise reasonable doubt about the presence of Alzheimer's or implicate other illnesses similar to Alzheimer's.[1] Early Alzheimer's disease needs to be reliably distinguished from normal aging.

## Medical Tests for Alzheimer's

As we talked about earlier, symptoms of delirium and Alzheimer's are shared by a number of other disorders. Once a good history is taken, the physician may order certain diagnostic medical tests.[2] The physician may look for neurological symptoms, review medications, check heart functioning, or check for brain wave abnormalities. The physician may test for thyroid functioning or a vitamin deficiency or ask for a urinalysis or order an imaging scan to rule out a stroke or tumor. For a more complete list of tests comprising a physician's standard workup for Alzheimer's, see appendix D, figure 2.

At some point in the assessment process, tests for mental status will be performed. Screening tests for mental status will usually be conducted by the family physician. More detailed tests for mental status will be completed by a psychologist. The general practice family physician may find it helpful to consult with a *geropsychologist* (a psychologist who specializes in the care of the elderly), a *neuropsychologist* (a psychologist specializing in the assessment of memory and other thinking functions), or other specialist who may have more training and experience working with dementia and other memory problems.

## Assessing for Delirium

Remember that as part of the process in assessing for Alzheimer's, it's essential to rule out the presence of delirium. One way to do that is through the *Confusion Assessment Method.*[3] A simple and straightforward measure of delirium, the Confusion Assessment Method is a handy tool to use when you suspect a person's thinking and behavior are unusual—even for them—and beyond what is typical or expected from Alzheimer's. The method identifies four symptomatic features of delirium:

> **Feature 1:** *Acute Onset*—The onset of the symptoms must be sudden (the change occurring over the course of 24 hours)
>
> **Feature 2:** *Inattention*—You see the person cannot focus or pay attention like they usually can. They are more easily distracted. Or they may have difficulty tracking what other people are saying. You test how attentive the person is by saying the following to them: "I am going to read you a series of letters. Just squeeze my hand when you hear the letter 'A,'" Then one-by-one, read each letter of a word like CASABLANCA—about 2–3 seconds apart. If they don't squeeze your hand after you call out an "A" or if they do squeeze your hand when you call out another letter, the person has made an error, and you can conclude Feature 2 is present.
>
> **Feature 3:** *Altered Level of Consciousness*—This feature is present when the person's level of arousal is anything other than calm and alert—that is, if they are combative, agitated, restless, drowsy, or sedated.
>
> **Feature 4:** *Disorganized Thinking*—This feature relates to how clear, organized, and logical the person's thinking is and is assessed by

asking the person the following YES/NO questions, all of which must be answered correctly:

◆ Will a stone float on water?

◆ Are there fish in the sea?

◆ Does one pound weigh more than two pounds?

◆ Can you use a hammer to pound a nail?

Delirium is present when:

Features 1 and 2 are present

AND

either Feature 3 or Feature 4 is present.

## Screening Tests for General Thinking Abilities

Abnormal cognitive functioning occurs in many illness and no more profoundly than in Alzheimer's. But many times, a thorough cognitive assessment is impractical or unnecessary. This is where screening methods are useful. There are a variety of ways to assess general thinking abilities and functioning, and they include the *Mini-Mental State Examination,* the *St. Louis University Mental Status Exam,* the *Montreal Cognitive Assessment,* and others.[4] Among the most informative are those that can detect skill deficits and strengths over a range of abilities. Depending on the clinician's level of training, the urgency needed to collect the information, and other factors, the clinician would choose which mental status tests would be the most appropriate for the particular circumstances.

**The Montreal Cognitive Assessment.** Let's first look at one of the most commonly used tests of mental capabilities—the Montreal Cognitive Assessment (MoCA). In the last chapter, we talked about Mary, who went into the hospital for hip surgery. Nowadays, she would likely be given the MoCA. The MoCA has been around since 2005 and is commonly used in hospital and other settings because it is free to use, quick to administer, sensitive to mild impairments in thinking, and available in different languages, and it provides the clinician with useful information on a person's overall thinking abilities. The MoCA measures eight principal areas of thought functioning:

1. *Visuospatial/Executive Functioning*—the person's ability to sequence, organize, and execute tracking a series of alphanumeric markers.

2. *Naming*—the person's ability to identify and name a series of animals.
3. *(Immediate) Memory*—the person's ability to store and immediately repeat a series of five words.
4. *Attention*—the person's ability to sustain attention to complete several alphanumeric tasks.
5. *Language*—the person's ability to read and draw upon their store of words.
6. *Abstraction*—the person's ability to conceptualize and abstract category labels from category examples.
7. *Delayed Recall*—the person's ability to recall words recited earlier in the test.
8. *Orientation*—the person's knowledge of the current date and location.

Several sample items comprising the MoCA are shown in figure 7a.[5] Scores on this assessment instrument range from 0 to 30. Scores of 26 and above are considered to be in the normal range. Scores of 19 to 25 are indicative of mild cognitive impairment. Scores of 21 and below may be indicative of Alzheimer's. As a screening tool, this test instrument is particularly sensitive and is now in wide use.

**Figure 7a.** Sample Items from the Montreal Cognitive Assessment

**Attention**
  ◆ Ask the person to subtract 7 from 100 and repeat subtracting from each new subtotal. Repeat five times.

**Language**
  ◆ Ask the person to name as many words as they can in 60 seconds that start with the letter F.

**Abstraction**
  ◆ Ask the person how a banana and an orange are alike. Repeat with two other examples.

**Delayed Recall**
  ◆ Ask the person to recall a list of five words they recited earlier in the test.

**Orientation**
  ◆ Ask the person the date, the month, the day, the year, and the city and place they are in.

*Adapted from the Montreal Cognitive Assessment (www.mocatest.org).*

Understanding the eight different aspects of functioning that comprise this instrument can help family members and other care providers become more mindful of what changes to look for as thinking abilities decline. Each of these thinking functions can be routinely monitored, and this can be an invaluable tool when communicating with other care providers on the person's mental status.

Although the MoCA is a quick and easy way to measure thinking abilities, the information it provides is limited. It's a screening tool and as such is not designed to be used in place of more thorough assessment methods. A tool like this should be used in the context of a periodic *Full Mental Status Exam*—a much more thorough and comprehensive assessment of both rational and irrational processes.

A Full Mental Status Exam would include an assessment of cognitive functioning but also an assessment of psychotic perceptions, mood and behavioral disturbances, defense mechanisms, coping styles, and other areas of psychological functioning. If you would like to learn more about what comprises a Full Mental Status Exam, take a look at appendix D, figure 3.

**The Clock Drawing Test.** While not originally developed to measure thinking functions in Alzheimer's, the *Clock Drawing Test* is another useful method and has been around for 50 years.[6] About 30 years ago, it was developed into a test instrument that captures many of the detriments in thinking exhibited by the Alzheimer's patient. Although it is a rather blunt instrument compared to more lengthy and sophisticated cognitive assessment methods, it is useful as a screening tool for clinicians to identify deficits that often manifest in Alzheimer's. Figure 7b shows how it works.

The patient is asked to draw a clock face, fill in the numbers, and draw the hands set to 10 minutes after 11:00. Once they do this, the drawing is scored for accuracy—usually by assigning

- – 1 point for drawing a circle,
- – 1 point for listing all 12 numbers,
- – 1 point for placing the numbers in the right order,
- – 1 point for drawing the two hands, and
- – 1 point for drawing the hands pointing to the correct time.

One or two mistakes are not indicative of Alzheimer's, but more than two mistakes often are. Figures 7c and 7d are clock drawings that were drawn by

**Figure 7b.** The Clock Drawing Test

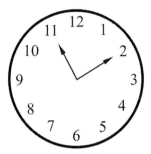

---

dementia patients with severe apraxia (trouble translating thoughts into actions). Figure 7e was drawn by a patient who had a stroke on the right side of their brain. Notice the neglect on the left side of the drawing. Shown in figure 7f is a drawing from someone who was taking a heart medication that the doctors were initially unaware was affecting their thinking abilities. Figure 7g shows a drawing from the same patient after their medication was switched. As I discussed in an earlier chapter, cognitive functioning deficits that look like Alzheimer's aren't always Alzheimer's.

## Screening Tests Specifically for Memory

There are many screening test instruments that are specific to measuring memory functioning. One of the simplest is the *Memory Impairment Screen.*[7] Here's how it works: The clinician chooses a word from each of four different

**Figure 7c.** Severe Apraxia

---

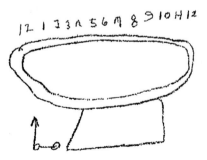

*Image courtesy of Brock et al., 1999.*

---

**Figure 7d.** Another Example of Severe Apraxia

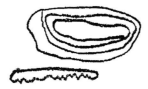

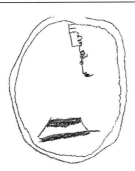

*Image courtesy of Brock et al., 1999.*

**Figure 7e.** A Clock Drawing from a Stroke Patient

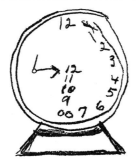

*Image courtesy of Joyce Shields.*

**Figure 7f.** A Medication Effect

*Image courtesy of Joyce Shields.*

**Figure 7g.** The Medication Effect Removed

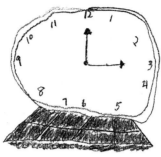

*Image courtesy of Joyce Shields.*

categories (e.g., vegetables, vehicles, clothing, and furniture), which is then printed in large capital letters on a piece of paper and given to the patient. The patient is then asked to read the four words aloud. I use the words CAR, CHAIR, SHIRT, and APPLE. After two or three minutes of conversing with them on another topic, the patient is asked to recall the four words. Two points are given for each word that is freely recalled. If needed, a category prompt is offered (for example, I might say, "One word was a fruit"), and one point is then given if they then can recall the word. Scores on the MIS range of 0–8, and a cutoff score of 4 or less is strongly indicative of dementia.

In another quick screening for memory problems, the person is shown and read the following name and address and asked to remember it:

"JOHN BROWN, 42 MARKET STREET, CHICAGO."

After a two-minute distraction task, one point is scored for each word remembered (the word STREET is not counted).[8] I usually distract them by asking them to complete the Clock Drawing Test. If they remember no more than two of the five countable words in the address, it may be indicative of memory impairment.

After I do this memory task and the Clock Drawing Test, I usually assess them for aphasia. Recall that in chapter 3, I discussed how aphasia (difficulty understanding or expressing language) is a hallmark sign in Alzheimer's— usually appearing in the earliest stages of the illness. Although there are more elaborate tests for identifying deficits in language, one of the easiest and quickest to administer is one of the screening tests for verbal fluency. I ask the person to imagine going to a grocery store, walking down the aisles, and

I then give them 60 seconds to name as many items as they can. A score of 7 items or less is indicative of dementia. But here's a neat little method of further interpretation: if the person also cannot remember more than two words from the John Brown address, *there is a 90 percent likelihood they are experiencing a dementia like Alzheimer's.*[9]

## More Thorough Psychological Tests for Alzheimer's

The clinician will often want more focused and specific ways to assess the deficits inherent in Alzheimer's disease, and several test instruments are available for this purpose. Two of the more common methods used to measure general dementia-related processes in Alzheimer's are the *Alzheimer's Disease Assessment Scale* and the *Dementia Rating Scale.*[10] The Dementia Rating Scale includes assessments for memory, aphasia, apraxia, executive functioning, and other thinking impairments indicative of Alzheimer's. It takes a psychologist about a half hour to administer the Dementia Rating Scale, and it provides a summary measure of skill deficits and strengths in the following five areas:

1. *Attention*—the ability to attend to verbal, visual, and numeric material;
2. *Initiation and Perseveration*—the ability to be verbally fluent and be persistent in carrying out verbal instructions;
3. *Construction*—the ability to copy and reproduce movements and visual designs;
4. *Conceptualization*—the ability to demonstrate higher-order executive reasoning; and
5. *Memory*—the ability to recall verbal and visual material.

Later on in this chapter, I provide an example of how the Dementia Rating Scale can be applied and interpreted, but it is important to note here that no single psychological test can be conclusive—no test can measure it all. Therefore, the clinician will need corroborating evidence on the presence and severity of any observed thinking impairments, and more specific tests to measure memory problems, word-finding difficulties, and other impairments in Alzheimer's are usually administered. One of the most common instruments used to assess memory impairments is the *Wechsler Memory Scale.*[11] Another instrument useful in assessing memory deficits in older adults is the *Kendrick Cognitive Test for the Elderly.*[12] The Wechsler Memory Scale is a well-established instrument, and its most recent version was developed from a sample of adults that included the elderly. The test takes a psychologist about an hour to administer and provides an accurate assessment of memory problems across several different memory domains, including visual and verbal memory, immediate recall of newly learned material, and attention and concentration processes in memory. This instrument also includes a measure of one area of memory considered to be among the most sensitive for detecting Alzheimer's—*delayed recall.* Here, the person is asked to recall information learned 20–30 minutes earlier.

To test specifically for deficits in language and symptoms of aphasia, a geropsychologist or neuropsychologist who is conducting a thorough neuropsychological assessment may use the *Boston Naming Test,* which detects problems in correctly naming common objects.[13] A test that is quite sensitive to impairments in executive functioning is called the *Wisconsin Card Sorting Test.*[14] The standard test battery I typically use includes the Dementia Rating Scale, the Wechsler Memory Scale, and often a general intelligence test like the *Wechsler Adult Intelligence Scale.*[15] Taken together with the results from the physician's observations, medical tests, and scans, these findings can pretty well determine the likely presence of Alzheimer's as well as the extent and severity of the illness.[16]

There also has been much written recently on how Alzheimer's seems to affect brain tissue governing the sense of smell. Researchers have found that people with cognitive impairments like Alzheimer's have a degraded sense of smell.[17] Although there is mounting evidence on the deficits in olfactory dysfunction in Alzheimer's and other neuropsychiatric illnesses, and hope for methods to eventually measure early olfactory biomarkers for these diseases, the research is still at a very early stage, and there is still no reliable way to diagnose Alzheimer's using a test of smelling abilities.

### *Roberta*

Roberta was a really neat lady. When I met her she was a 76-year-old African American woman, widowed, and recently admitted to an extended care facility, and I was asked by a regional social service agency to conduct a competency evaluation. She was briefly hospitalized prior to coming to the facility because of severe memory problems, rapid and rambling speech, and a long and recently exacerbated history of behavioral problems in her apartment building, including: the conviction that her neighbors were invading her apartment and stealing her food, the belief that her deceased parents were still alive and for whom Roberta had been putting out food, and the perception that her deceased brother was still alive and was tripping and pushing her. Chart records also indicated that over the years when she was living in the community, there were periods when Roberta refused to take her prescribed psychiatric mediations. Earlier that year, though, she was living at home, taking her medications, and was reportedly managing her psychiatric symptoms just fine.

Roberta was interviewed in her wheelchair, but she was receiving physical therapy where they were helping her walk without assistance. She was, nonetheless, currently at risk for falls. She had some trouble with bladder incontinence and was also diagnosed with congestive heart failure and hypertension. When I talked with Roberta she was alert, very polite and cooperative, knew who she was and where she was, and was in good spirits—absent any of the elevated mood, psychotic symptoms, and problematic behaviors that precipitated her hospital admission. She had a quiet sophistication and calmness to her demeanor—as if she were merely humoring me by cooperating with my evaluation. At the same time, she radiated a knowing optimism that seemed to convey that everything would turn out just fine for her. It was apparent, however, that despite her denials, Roberta had severe short-term memory problems. She also denied the multiple psychiatric hospitalizations of record or ever having taken psychiatric medications prior to her nursing home admission. Her current medication regimen included Lasix (a medicine used to treat hypertension and congestive heart failure), Aricept (an anti-dementia medication), Depakote (a mood stabilizer), Zoloft (an antidepressant), and Risperdal (an antipsychotic), all of which I will discuss in more detail in chapter 12. There was nothing particularly remarkable about her social history or background—she had been married twice but had no children and had a bachelor's degree upon which she built a long and successful professional career.

About a month prior to my interview with her, Roberta scored 20 out of 30 on the Mini-Mental State Examination, and I administered the *Hopkins Competency Test* (which I will talk a little more about in chapter 9) and the Dementia Rating Scale. Her test results for the Dementia Rating Scale are shown in table 7a, and as you can see, her total score on this measurement instrument indicated the presence of dementia. If you look carefully at the five subscales comprising that score, though, only one of them, "Memory," is indicative of dementia—the rest of them were considered all within the normal range. Her memory score was so poor, however, that it pulled the total score

**Table 7a.** Roberta's Scores on the Dementia Rating Scale

| Scale | Raw Score | Above/Below Cutoff Indicative of Dementia |
|---|---|---|
| DRS Total Score | 118 | Below (indicative) |
| Memory | 11 | Below (indicative) |
| Attention | 36 | Above (not indicative) |
| Initiation and Perseveration | 32 | Above (not indicative) |
| Construction | 5 | Above (not indicative) |
| Conceptualization | 34 | Above (not indicative) |

in the range indicative of dementia, but there appeared to be no serious deficits in other areas of cognitive functioning—something that is necessary for a diagnosis of Alzheimer's. This set of scores would indicate mild cognitive impairment and not dementia. On the Hopkins Competency Assessment Test (discussed in detail in chapter 8), Roberta scored a 5 out of 10, which is above the threshold for competency and thus indicated that Roberta was most likely competent to make her own medical decisions.

I believe that Roberta had mild cognitive impairment—not dementia—and bipolar disorder (something I will talk more about in chapter 12). She had severe short-term memory problems but no other significant cognitive deficits, and I believe that, at the time of the evaluation, Roberta was competent to make her own medical decisions. That being said, however, it certainly appeared that Roberta had the precursor symptoms of Alzheimer's, and because she had a history of poor medication compliance, it seemed likely she was bound to repeat her noncompliant medication pattern in the future, especially given her memory problems. Recall also from chapter 1 that the conversion rate from mild cognitive impairment to a bona fide diagnosis of Alzheimer's is about 15–20 percent per year. Given all this, I recommended that a guardian of person and property be assigned who could work with Roberta to protect her from harm while helping her maintain as independent a lifestyle as possible and offering her the widest possible latitude in choosing where she wanted to live—in essence, a kind of limited and individualized guardianship. Supportive counseling, more intensive home assistance, and the involvement of the local Council on Aging were all things I believed would also be helpful for her.

Helping someone through an assessment process for Alzheimer's can feel like a daunting task. It can frighten, frustrate, and discourage the person being assessed, not to mention her family members. Once through it, though, the needed advice and assistance can then be made available. It is at this point that at least some of the uncertainty of the present can evaporate into possibilities and clarity about the future.

# 8

# Measuring Alzheimer's in Action

"Accidents, injury, and sickness are strong
and loving ways in which the Universe gets
your undivided attention."[1]

## The Global Deterioration Scale

In the process of making a diagnosis of Alzheimer's, the extent, severity, and progression of the illness is always assessed. Researchers have developed several ways of thinking about the level of impairment of the elderly person with Alzheimer's.[2] One method employs what's called the *Global Deterioration Scale* (see figure 8a), which helps the clinician get a better picture of how far the disease has progressed. Seven levels of severity are categorized.

### *Level 1: No Cognitive Decline (Optimal Functioning)*
This level indicates no complaints or problems in memory or thinking.

### *Level 2: Very Mild Cognitive Decline (Common Forgetfulness)*
This level indicates slight problems in memory but no more than would be

**Figure 8a.** The Global Deterioration Scale

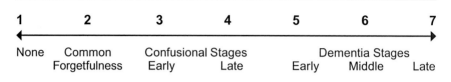

considered normal—for example, forgetting where you put your car keys, briefly forgetting the name of someone you know. If a clinical interview was conducted or a psychological assessment instrument was administered, the results would show nothing significant. At this very mild level of severity, people will show appropriate concern for any memory problems they might have.

### Level 3: Mild Cognitive Decline (Early Confusional Stage)

It is at this level that thinking problems become more noticeable and provide an early indication of cognitive decline. To qualify for this mild level of severity, the person must exhibit at least two of the following symptoms:

- ◆ The person will often get lost while traveling to a familiar location. For example, I've had clients who have told me, "I lived here for many years, and I am getting lost more and more now. I just drive around until I find something familiar or call home."
- ◆ Word-finding or naming difficulties become more obvious to those who know the person well. The person might reflect on his cognitive decline by saying, "I don't like being around people now because I mess up what I want to say," or he might say, "I know what I want to say but it just comes out wrong." The person might also begin substituting one word for another, for example, "wet" for "water" or "opening" for "door."
- ◆ The person can't remember much of what he may have just read.
- ◆ The names of people newly introduced are quickly forgotten.
- ◆ The person repeatedly loses his wallet, ring, keys, or other things of value.
- ◆ Concentration and memory deficits become more prominent. For example, the person might tell you, "I have a hard time staying focused or making decisions." People at work or at home begin to notice something is wrong with the person's thinking or memory, and when formally and professionally assessed memory problems are more

clearly identified. Despite what others see, the person may actually believe he does not have a problem.

◆ Mild anxiety or depression may also begin to appear. Clients have told me, "I go to the doctor's, but mostly I'm afraid to go out, so I just wind up staying home alone."

### *Level 4: Moderate Cognitive Decline (Late Confusional Stage)*

At this moderate stage of the disease, the person's orientation to the date or time is usually normal. The severity of problems, however, becomes more clear-cut to others and may manifest in the following ways:

◆ The person's knowledge of current or recent events becomes poor.

◆ The person begins to have difficulty remembering parts of his own personal history.

◆ Difficulties arise when trying to count backwards from 100 by 7's or by 3's or when trying to spell the word "WORLD" backwards.

◆ The person's ability to travel, handle finances, or complete other complex tasks is significantly diminished.

◆ Out of embarrassment or the inability to accept what he is experiencing, the person may deny having any memory problems.

◆ Depressed mood and a kind of emotional dullness pervade the person's experience.

◆ The person has a greater tendency to avoid situations that challenge him.

### *Level 5: Moderately Severe Cognitive Decline (Early Dementia)*

At this moderately severe level, the person is no longer able to manage her affairs on her own and needs assistance from others. She can remember her own name, the name of her spouse, or the names of her children, and can still conduct certain daily chores in her routine, like toileting or eating, but she is more likely to have trouble picking out appropriate clothing or putting it on correctly. She also has problems with the following:

◆ The person may have difficulty remembering her address or her long-time telephone number. She may also have trouble remembering her grandchildren's names or have difficulty recalling significant personal information about her history, like where she went to high school.

◆ She is frequently disoriented to the date, the day of the week, the season, or the name of the town where she has lived.

- Someone with a good education may, nonetheless, have trouble counting backwards from 20 by 4's or by 2's.
- Mood problems get worse.

## Level 6: Severe Cognitive Decline (Middle Dementia)

The disease is quite severe at this stage. The person will almost always be able to recall her own name, and she is usually able to recognize familiar people and locations, but she may forget the name of her spouse or may not be aware of any recent events or experiences in her life. Her memory of her own life is usually very poor, and she may not know what year or season it is. In addition, the following characteristics may also be evident:

- The person is not able to count backwards from 10 to 1 or, sometimes, even forwards from 1 to 10.
- She is frequently incontinent.
- Emotional problems become more severe—for example, the person may believe her spouse is an impostor or she may talk to her reflection in the mirror. She may repeat phrases or simple actions, like repeatedly cleaning something. Her level of anxiety and agitation increases and aggressive behavior may begin to emerge. The person may also lose her ability to make simple decisions or exercise her free will.

## Level 7: Very Severe Cognitive Decline (Late Dementia)

This is the worst stage of the disease. At this point, the person is having severe difficulty forming any words at all, and he is totally dependent on others for toileting and feeding himself. He cannot coordinate his muscles to walk, and his brain is no longer able to communicate with the rest of his body to carry out purposeful action.

To better understand the early regressive stages of the Alzheimer's sufferer, I would like to make an analogy to the development of the growing child. We know that kids develop though certain predictable stages. By the time they are two years old, kids are beginning to learn how to organize their world and direct and coordinate their own actions. By the time they are seven, they can attend to several factors at the same time and sort out information they deem irrelevant to decision making. They also begin to develop the ability to take another person's point of view. By age ten, although able to understand abstract rules like "Good rest and good eating habits are important," the thinking processes of the ten-year-old are still very concrete. Their ability to embrace the possible, the hypothetical, and potential cause-and-effect relationships, as grown adults do, is still underdeveloped. Just as children *progress* through predicable and identifiable stages, people with Alzheimer's *regress* through similar stages.

Let's use this analogy so we might better understand, for example, why someone with Alzheimer's might leave the stove on. He may not only have forgotten to turn it off, but he might not have been as able to abstractly conceptualize the idea that lit stoves can cause fires. He may be more stubborn and defensive when hearing that he left the stove on because he may be having more difficulty taking another person's point of view. The following quote from Elizabeth Cohen's poignant account of her husband's battle with Alzheimer's nicely illustrates the analogy with the growing child.

> Ava learns to walk and talk while Sanford forgets how to climb stairs and struggles with his vocabulary (when he can't remember the word "water," he substitutes "the liquid substance from the spigot"). Daddy walks around now this way, dropping pieces of language behind him, the baby following, picking them up.[3]

Clinicians have long used a person's ability to copy a drawing of a clock as a rough tool in assessing the cognitive abilities of people who have suffered a brain injury. Researchers have now innovatively applied this tool to measure cognitive abilities in Alzheimer's patients. They found that the thinking skills needed to copy a picture of a clock inversely correlates with the person's level of cognitive deterioration as measured by the Global Deterioration Scale—that is, the poorer his score on the Clock Drawing Test, the higher his level of severity on the Global Deterioration Scale.[4] Researchers are also exploring the extent to which deterioration in Alzheimer's inversely correlates with common measures of childhood development. Based on this research, an activity program geared to the particular cognitive abilities of the Alzheimer's patient has been designed, and I will discuss more about this in chapter 15.

## Functional Abilities

To say someone has memory and thinking problems does not necessarily say much about how well he carries out his day-to-day life activities. As I have discussed, Alzheimer's affects thinking, emotion and perceptions, and functional capabilities. Ironically, neuropsychological tests of memory, language comprehension and production, and other cognitive functions don't reliably predict how well a person will function in the "real world." Therefore, a thorough assessment for Alzheimer's disease must include measures of *functional ability*. Figure 8b illustrates how functional abilities vary in complexity and can be ranked in terms of the mental capacity needed to accomplish them.[5]

As I've mentioned, when a person with Alzheimer's begins to lose his functional abilities, the telltale signs are often detected first by family, friends, or coworkers—that is, by those with whom the person is the closest or has the most contact. In their ranking, social roles and skilled performance levels are considered to be the most cognitively complex tasks and are the most likely to reveal deficits first. As Alzheimer's progresses, the person will first begin to lose the ability to effectively manage his job, relationships, and finances; his ability to drive and to prepare meals; and his ability to properly manage other *instrumental* (advanced) *activities of daily living* (IADLs). These activities are essential for effective social or occupational functioning. As the disease progresses, the person's ability to maintain proper grooming, dressing, and other basic *activities of daily living* (ADLs) then becomes compromised.

Researchers have provided some useful ways of thinking about and measuring functional competencies in elderly people, and one assessment scale particularly sensitive to changes in ADLs and IADLs across the progressive phases of Alzheimer's disease is called the *Direct Assessment of Functional Status*.[6] Another assessment instrument commonly used to measure functional abilities is called the *Community Competency Scale*.[7] Each of these instruments includes ways to measure the following abilities:

- ◆ To access and use transportation
- ◆ To see, hear, and touch clearly and accurately
- ◆ To maintain a household
- ◆ To walk or wheel around
- ◆ To maintain personal hygiene
- ◆ To wear clean clothes and do laundry
- ◆ To prepare a shopping list and purchase the items
- ◆ To manage finances
- ◆ To use the telephone
- ◆ To communicate clearly with others
- ◆ To prepare meals and maintain a proper diet
- ◆ To handle emergencies
- ◆ To care for one's own medical needs
- ◆ To compensate for one's own deficits

**Figure 8b.** A Hierarchical Model of Functional Abilities

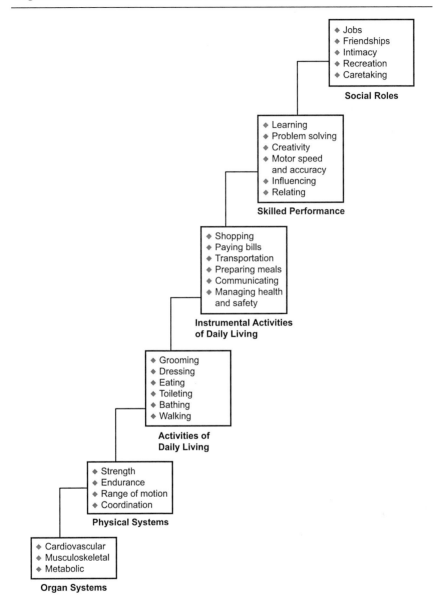

Taken from Kemp and Mitchell (1992). Used with permission.

*The Interview for Deterioration in Daily Living Activities in Dementia* is another commonly used test instrument—this one targeting lower level functional abilities, such as the person's ability to wash themselves, make coffee or tea, dress themselves, and so forth.[8] Once a functional assessment has been completed, the clinician will have a better idea of the progression of the disease and the level of competency the person possesses to cope with the disease.

Jean Piaget was a Swiss psychologist who was instrumental in helping us understand how thinking develops in kids, and his perspective can help us further understand the progression of Alzheimer's. Piaget showed us that thinking in children progresses in several stages, where the child develops more and more sophisticated ways of thinking about themselves and the world. In chapter 3, I told you a story of how Charlotte paraded in her home like a glorious bride and how her thinking had regressed to that of a child. Well, you can think of the regression in thinking in Alzheimer's as the opposite of the progression in thinking that Piaget spoke about. So, if you overlay the Global Deterioration Scale discussed earlier in this chapter, the scores on the Clock Drawing Test (discussed in chapter 7), the hierarchical levels of functional abilities (discussed earlier in this chapter), and Piaget's age-associated stages of cognitive development, a deeper and more detailed picture of the degeneration in Alzheimer's begins to appear. These comparisons appear in figure 8c.

**Figure 8c.** Comparing Perspectives in the Progression of Alzheimer's

*Global Deterioration Scale*

| 1 | 2 | 3 | 4 | 5 | 6 | 7 |
|---|---|---|---|---|---|---|

None — Common Forgetfulness — Confusional Stages (Early, Late) — Dementia Stages (Early, Middle, Late)

| Global Deterioration Scale | Clock Drawing Test | Levels of Functional Abilities* | Piagetian Stages of Childhood Development |
|:---:|:---:|:---:|:---:|
| 1 | 5 out of 5 | No impairments | 10 or older |
| 2 | 5 out of 5 | No impairments | 10 or older |
| 3 | 5 out of 5 | Social roles | 10 or older |
| 4 | 4 out of 5 | Skilled performance | 10 or older |
| 5 | 3 out of 5 | IADLs | 7–10 |
| 6 | 1 or 2 out of 5 | ADLs | 2–7 |
| 7 | 0 or 1 out of 5 | Physical systems | 0–2 |

*Social roles, skilled performance, IADLs, ADLs, physical systems.

People in the normal range on the Global Deterioration Scale tend to do well on the Clock Drawing Test; they also do well in executing their social roles until their illness progresses to the confusional stage, where they begin to show signs of the illness. A Clock Drawing Test score of 3 out of 5 seems to correspond to the early to middle dementia stage of progression, where the person may show signs of the illness in their IADLs. They may then begin to act and think in ways that have regressed to approximately the cognitive development of a seven- to ten-year-old. As the disease progresses further into the middle and late dementia stages, their clock drawing scores diminish, they are having more trouble with their ADLs and with strength and coordination (the physical systems), and their thinking regresses to earlier and earlier stages of childhood.

Understanding that Alzheimer's is a progressive, debilitating illness can be emotionally crippling to those who suffer with it and to those who see it. Coming to grips with and truly accepting the undeniable fact that life has suffering paradoxically nourishes the belief that there is a larger and loving Universe out there—one with its own plan and its own design for all of us. Alzheimer's is a reminder to us that what we do not understand can teach us something about ourselves, our lives, and the lives of others. To resist life's natural currents is like swimming upstream. Instead, flow with it.

# 9

# The Question of Competence

> "Imagine that every person in the world is enlightened but you. They are all your teachers, each doing just the right things to help you learn perfect patience, perfect wisdom, perfect compassion."

Enid is 86 years old and lives alone, and she was about to incur a high cost for repairs on her home. Enid's children are concerned about their mother's decision-making ability and want to make themselves their mother's power of attorney. So, they take Enid to a local attorney for a consultation. The lawyer is a friend of yours and has never consulted anyone on this issue before. They know, though, that you have been reading up on Alzheimer's and call you for some advice. What do you tell the attorney?

Your neighbor, Andrew, and his son have lived next door to you for many years. Andrew just turned 75 and had been in a terrible car accident but has just received a large insurance settlement. He wants to use the money to travel overseas. But when his son takes Andrew to the doctor for a routine follow-up appointment, the doctor notices some thinking changes in Andrew, pulls his son aside, and tells him that he should think about seeking guardianship of his father. In a tizzy, the son calls you. What do you say to the son?

Aunt Berty is 81, and her primary care physician feels she can't think for herself and refers her for a "competency evaluation." You are Aunt Berty's favorite relative and learn that her physician called her competence into question because she refused to follow his advice to undergo a procedure for a corneal implant. Aunt Berty calls you and asks you what she should do.

The Bertys, the Andrews, and the Enids of the world struggle with issues like these every day, and those involved in their care have badly needed informed advice about what should be done for them. More than any other group, the issue of functional competence is central to the lives of the Alzheimer's family. Alzheimer's families are often troubled by such questions as "Can my parent live alone?" "How much supervision does he need?" "Will he be safe on his own?" and "Can she handle her own affairs?" It's usually the children (most often daughters) of the Alzheimer's sufferer who wrestle most with these difficult issues. What I am talking about here is the issue of whether a person has the capacities necessary to be trusted with their own decision making. For those questioning someone's capacity to make sound decisions, the core dilemma centers around two conflicting values: (1) the duty to protect the person from making decisions that could be potentially harmful to themselves or others, and (2) the responsibility to honor the person's right to their own self-determination.[1]

Competence is a legal term, and there are a wide variety of legal competencies. For example:

◆ a person's competence to stand trial might be questioned;
◆ a person's competency to waive their rights of silence or of legal counsel—so-called Miranda rights;
◆ someone's competency to assume criminal responsibility for a crime might be questioned—for example, being deemed "not guilty by reason of insanity";
◆ a parent's competency to take legal custody of their child might be in doubt; and
◆ a person's competence to consent to participate in a research study might be questioned.

But when it comes to Alzheimer's dementia the most frequent matters of competency relate to

◆ a person's capacity for caring for themselves or their property; or
◆ a person's capacity to consent to medical treatment.

The terms most associated with the first issue are *guardianship* or *conservatorship,* and the term most associated with the latter issue is *informed consent.*

Fully addressing questions of legal capacity for sound decision making is a complicated matter.[2] What you should know, however, is that the process usually begins with a petition to the court, either by a family member or by a qualified clinician. Information provided by family members can be very important in the assessment process, but a clinician's thorough evaluation should always include a complete mental status evaluation of the person along with psychological testing. Family physicians can provide the court with some of the evidence needed for the determination of a person's capacity, but in most situations, a judge or general physician will consult someone with more specialized training and experience in assessing cognitive capacity in older adults. The key questions the clinician and the court should be addressing are as follows:

1. Does the person have the capacity to understand and comprehend the choice that is before them?
2. Does the person have the capacity to communicate and express their choice in terms of what they want and need?
3. Does the person have the insight and foresight to appreciate the benefits and risks of their choice?
4. Does the person have the capacity to reason through and explain the logic or rationale behind their choice?[3]

In order for a court to consider whether a person is legally competent to make her own financial and medical decisions, the clinician must submit a "Statement of Expert Evaluation." This is a short document—usually created in the appropriate local municipality outlining the following information:

1. A diagnosis of the person's mental incapacity;
2. Evidence to support the diagnosis of mental incapacity;
3. The identified cause of the mental incapacity; and
4. An opinion about the person's ability to conduct business affairs or make competent medical decisions without the aid of someone else (a guardian).

However, this document is a very short summary of the clinician's general findings and should never be submitted by a physician or other qualified professional as a standalone document—that is, to be a thorough and complete submission to the court, the Statement of Expert Evaluation should be accompanied by an exhaustive report covering, in detail, all the information the judge needs to render an informed decision. Unfortunately, this is not always the case.

Before we go any further with our discussion of capacity, I want to provide you with a little historical background. Before 1980, the basic protocol for the evaluation of mental capacity was limited to the following:

◆ A medical doctor or psychiatrist or other state authorized clinician (usually a psychologist or licensed social worker) examined the patient.
◆ The authorized clinician made a diagnosis.
◆ A judge was petitioned and reached a judicial opinion that was often based on the diagnosis alone.

For example, if the patient was diagnosed with dementia the judge would often deem the patient incompetent to manage their own affairs—that is, the judge's decision was based on the diagnosis alone. In 85 percent of the cases, the person who was the subject of the legal matter was not even present in the courtroom. In only 3 percent of the cases was the person, whose capacity was being questioned, represented by council. The hearings usually lasted just a few minutes. And the petitions for guardianship—the document that begins the process—were denied in only about 4 percent of the cases![4] Quite often in these cases, family members, clinicians, and judges all made erroneous summary judgments about a person's capacity by giving more weight to the person's choice (e.g., to avoid a costly or risky medical procedure) than to the process the person used to arrive at that choice. Courts often assumed that a person who lacked capacity for one type of decision also must lack the capacity for all other types of decisions.[5]

Too often still today, many judges base their conclusions of competency on the presence of emotional or behavioral dyscontrol. However, a determination of incompetency cannot be predominantly and sufficiently based on issues of behavioral or emotional dyscontrol. Here's an example of what I mean: an under-medicated schizophrenic or a binging alcoholic can certainly manifest behaviors and emotions that would be considered inadequately controlled, but that person cannot be considered permanently and legally incompetent to make medical and financial decisions unless treatment options to remedy the dyscontrol are first explored and the cause of the aberrant behavior is determined to be intractable. Some medications can help Alzheimer's patients regain emotional control just as they would likely help an under-medicated schizophrenic.

Studies evaluating guardianship protocols after 1980 have shown that the attendance of the person in question increased to about 28 percent. In 25 percent of these cases, the person is now being represented by an attorney. But quite often, the attorney is unclear about the role to be played. Their confusion centers around the degree to which they see themselves as their client's advocate regardless of the client's mental state or whether they see their role as looking out for their client's safety.[6]

The clinician helps the court decide issues of capacity by rendering a professional opinion to the judge, but it's the judge who actually decides whether a person is competent or not. The American Psychological Association and the American Bar Association got together and developed best practice standards to help both the clinician and the judge.[7] Whether you are a lawyer, a physician, a psychiatrist, a psychologist, Enid's friend, Andrew's next-door neighbor, or Berty's niece or nephew, it is important to understand the process of assessing the decision-making capacity of an older adult. Here's what the APA and the ABA proposed.

Current "best practice" protocols call for the clinician to do much more than merely diagnose the patient. They call for the clinician to

- ◆ interview the patient, their family, and those professionals who are caring for the patient;
- ◆ evaluate the thinking ability, emotional state, perceptions, and behaviors of the patient;
- ◆ assess the patient's values, goals, and preferences; and
- ◆ evaluate the *functional capacity* of the patient—that is, to assess what functions the patient is able to perform and what functions they are not able to perform.

This last aspect of the clinician's evaluation tries to address what functional capacity of the patient is actually in question—for example, are people worried about the person's ability to drive, make a wise choice to marry, consent to have sex with their choice of partner, execute advanced directives, consent to medical care, write checks, sell property, enter into a contract, manage a large financial portfolio, what? Despite the ABA and APA recommendations proposed, this functional aspect of a proper capacity evaluation is sorely absent in most capacity determinations today. You might not be aware of this, but

76 percent of drivers with mild Alzheimer's can pass a Department of Motor Vehicles driving test.[8]

Not to complicate matters, but each state has its own definition of "competence." Most legal definitions of competence for self-guardianship include a phrase such as "incapable of taking proper care of himself, his property, or other persons for whom he is charged to provide." Some states are quite detailed in their definition; others are not; some states are very strict in their definition; others are more lenient. This variance has been confusing and has led to the development of what's called the Uniform Probate Code (written by the National Conference of Commissioners on Uniform State Laws), which attempts to draw national standards that can make more consistent the way the various legal systems across the country regard mental capacity.[9]

This brings us to the notion of exactly what it means to be fair about these pronouncements of thinking capacity—that is, what it means to make a fair legal judgment about another person's mental capacity. The words of forensic psychologist Thomas Grisso and forensic psychiatrist Paul Appelbaum ring true here:

> The right of capable persons to make their own decisions about their medical, financial, and life issues is at the foundation of the American legal system and the basis for ethical clinical practice.[10]

> How much of a deficit in abilities is enough to justify the restriction of individual liberties . . . requires a moral and social judgment, not a scientific or clinical one.[11]

Fairly judging a person's capacity requires honoring their right to make what others might feel is a "wrong" decision. For me, the most difficult part of doing a capacity evaluation centers on answering this question: How much should a person be allowed to make his own *bad* decision without interference from others? Every parent of a budding teenager knows this dilemma, and the conflict is similar when evaluating the competence of someone with Alzheimer's. Clinicians generally agree that the right to make a bad decision can be denied only when it can be stated with some degree of certainty that the person does not have the capacity to fully understand his choices. If there is sufficient evidence to support that a person with Alzheimer's cannot comprehend the implications of their decisions, then the clinician should conclude that the person is not competent to make those choices on their own.

What the clinician, the judge, and family members are all trying to do is to balance the person's need to be protected from harm while honoring the person's fundamental need for autonomy and self-determination. In a criminal trial, the judge or jury uses the decision rule "proof beyond a reasonable doubt." In many states, the judge decides if the person is competent to the task that is relevant—for example, making medical decisions, living on their own, spending money as they choose—by employing a decision rule that is based on the "preponderance of proof." This means that the judge's decision is based on what 51 percent of the evidence implies. In some states, the law requires a judge to render their decision based on "clear and convincing evidence"—based on what roughly 75 percent of the evidence shows.

## The Six Pillars of a Capacity Assessment

The American Bar Association, the American Psychological Association, and the National College of Probate Judges developed some important guidelines for judges to make the complex and frequently heart-wrenching decisions around thinking capacity.[12] They concluded that a competently performed capacity assessment should address the following:

1. *The person's medical condition:*
   - ◆ What is the medical condition affecting the person's functioning?
   - ◆ What is the history of the condition?
   - ◆ How severe is the condition?
   - ◆ Will the condition improve with time or treatment?
   - ◆ What are any reversible or mitigating factors affecting the condition?
2. *The person's thinking abilities, their mood, and the intensity of their emotions:*
   - ◆ How alert and attentive is the person?
   - ◆ How well do they process new information?
   - ◆ Are there obsessions, compulsions, phobias, hallucinations, or delusions?
   - ◆ How well is the person able to manage their emotions?
3. *The person's everyday functioning:* This relates to the hierarchy of functional abilities shown in chapter 8 in figure 8a. You can think of functional deterioration in terms of movement down the hierarchy to less and less sophisticated levels of functioning and mental capacity or "competence" in terms of movement up the hierarchy.

4. *The consistency of the person's choices and their values and preferences:*
   ◆ Does the person want a guardian? If so, who would it be?
   ◆ How does the person want to make important decisions—alone or with help from others?
   ◆ Where do they want to live? Why?
   ◆ What makes life meaningful or good for them?
   ◆ What activities are the most important to them?
   ◆ Does their religion play a role in how their decisions are made?

5. *The person's risk of harm and the level of supervision that may be needed:*
   ◆ What are the risks the person is currently facing?
   ◆ How do their relationships with others protect them from or enhance those risks?
   ◆ How significant are the risks? How likely are the risks to occur?
   ◆ How much supervision is needed to ensure the person's safety while preserving their sense of autonomy?

6. *The means available to the person to enhance their functioning:* This addresses whether there are treatments or accommodations that might enhance or restore the person's functioning.

Once the assessing clinician addresses these questions, the information is then passed on to the judge. In arriving at a determination of capacity, the ABA, APA, and NCPJ suggest that the judge take on a more nuanced and enlightened role than ever before. As they put it:

> Judges are not like baseball umpires calling strikes and balls or merely labeling someone competent or incompetent. Rather the better analogy is that of a craftsman who carves staffs from tree branches.[13]

Judges are advised to try to balance multiple goals by honoring the person's well-being and rights, by providing guidance to guardians, by being mindful of methods of restoration when possible, and by identifying the *least restrictive alternative* to guardianship. According to the Uniform Probate Code:

> Like other areas of the law where the concept of capacity is used, the required incapacity for the appointment of a guardian is no longer

considered an all-or-nothing proposition but instead it is recognized as having varying degrees. . . . This definition is designed to work with the concepts of least restrictive alternative and limited guardianship or conservatorship—only removing those rights that the incapacitated person cannot exercise, and not establishing a guardianship or conservatorship if a lesser restrictive alternative exists.[14]

As of July 2016, the following states have adopted the Uniform Probate Code guidelines for limited guardianships: Alaska, Arizona, Colorado, Florida, Hawaii, Idaho, Maine, Massachusetts, Michigan, Minnesota, Montana, Nebraska, New Mexico, North Dakota, South Carolina, South Dakota, and Utah. Other states have adopted the UPC guidelines in a less complete form. Shown in table 9a are examples of less restrictive alternatives to guardianship.[15]

Most of the time, the courts assign a guardian for financial decisions, healthcare decisions, or both. In many jurisdictions, though, the court has the flexibility to assign a guardian with only limited authority in specific areas or to assign someone who has general authority for making decisions on the person's behalf. This would depend on the court's judgment of the person's functional abilities. As we described in the last chapter, functional abilities can be measured on different levels. For example, a person may have the ability to maintain personal hygiene or care for their living space, but may be unable to manage their own finances or think through common emergencies. You can see, then, that how much autonomy the court grants a person depends on the nature and potential implications of the decisions they would be faced to make.

In what's called a *limited guardianship,* the individual might retain the right to determine their own living arrangements, spend small amounts of money, make and communicate choices about who they want to live with, initiate and follow a schedule of daily or leisure activities, establish and maintain personal relationships with whom they choose, or determine their degree of participation in religious activities. Earlier in the book, I told you about my client, Michael. He was assigned a guardian whose power was limited to managing his general finances, but Michael was granted the right to write checks to his local grocery store on his own.

Ultimately, the judge has the job to pull together all the information they have gathered and draw a conclusion about the thinking capacity of a person. When they do this with prudence and thoroughness, they must consider the person's abilities relative to the demands being made on them. The judge also

**Table 9a.** Less Restrictive Alternatives to Guardianship

| Category | Tasks | Social Services | Legal Mechanisms |
|---|---|---|---|
| Finances | Managing assets<br>Paying bills<br>Writing a will | Bill paying services<br>Money management services | Conservatorship<br>Representative Payee<br>Trustee<br>Durable power of attorney<br>Healthcare proxy |
| Health | Medical decision making<br>Healthcare/ medication management | Visiting nurse<br>Pill box/dispensing systems<br>Telephone reminder systems | Power of attorney<br>Healthcare proxy |
| Independent living | Household cleaning<br>Laundry<br>Shopping<br>Meal preparation<br>Personal hygiene | Emergency call systems<br>Meals on Wheels<br>Life Alert<br>Home health aide<br>Assisted living | None noted |
| Transportation | Driving<br>Use of public transportation | Driver training<br>Rides to appointments<br>Assists with public transportation | Driver testing |

Taken from Moye (2003). Used with permission.

weighs the potential benefits of guardianship over the harm it could cause. Here, the judge is trying to balance overall gains and risks. When the risks for harm without a guardian are high and the benefits of assigning one are high, the decision to assign a guardian is less pondering. Likewise, when the risks for harm are low and other means to assist the person in their decision making are available, the easier the judgment becomes.

There are many test instruments available to assess overall capacity to make independently and autonomously sound medical and other life decisions. Two of the most commonly administered are the *Hopkins Capacity Assessment Test*[16] and the *MacArthur Competence Assessment Tool for Treatment* (MacCAT-T).[17] The Hopkins Competency Assessment Test takes about 10 minutes to administer and begins by first reading to the person a set of short paragraphs that include information about medical decision making, power of attorney, and how a person's thinking can deteriorate in the course of a debilitating illness. After the paragraphs are read aloud, a series of questions are posed, and the person's responses are then scored and tallied. I have included the questions and answers used in this measurement instrument in appendix D, figure 4. This assessment tool is quite reliable and accurately predicts what a judge might decide about a person's capacity to make sound medical decisions.

The MacCAT-T is a structured interview that takes about 20 minutes to administer. It is tailored to the patient and is designed to assess and incorporate their particular medical information. The patient's responses are evaluated as either adequate, partial, or inadequate in each of three areas of ability: (1) how well they understand the medical decision facing them, (2) how well they have reasoned through their decision, and (3) how well they can appreciate the gravity of their decision. Unlike the Hopkins Competency Assessment Test, the MacCAT-T is intended to measure relative abilities in the three specific areas just mentioned but is not designed to provide an overall measure of competence. The ability-specific results from the MacCAT-T are interpreted in light of other relevant clinical information.

## The Case of Jackie Daniels

I once conducted a capacity evaluation on a 78-year-old never married, retired Euro-American woman who was living on a locked dementia unit in an assisted living facility. The court asked me to conduct the evaluation after the family had asked for a transfer of guardianship to a different family member.

Four years prior, Jackie was living an independent life with her sister; then her sister died. Two years later, Jackie lost her way driving and called a family member for help. When they took Jackie home they found it in disarray—broken glass, cigarette burns, a neglected dog, and Post-it notes everywhere. The family then arranged for her relocation to an assisted living facility—a decision with which Jackie initially agreed. Upon admission to the facility, Jackie was diagnosed with Alcohol Induced Dementia, soon after became quite surly, and was subsequently evaluated by a local psychiatrist, who asserted that Jackie was unable to manage her own affairs. The psychiatrist and family petitioned the court, and Jackie was deemed incompetent to manage her own affairs.

Jackie had a bachelor's degree in education, a 25-year history in teaching, but a lifelong struggle with alcohol abuse, which was patently evident to her family but which she chronically denied. She had no other medical issues. When I went to the facility to evaluate her she was friendly and cooperative, fluent and detailed in her speech, and had no observable signs of apraxia, agnosia, or deficits in executive functioning—symptoms besides memory loss needed for any diagnosis of dementia. The facility staff reported that her Activities of Daily Living were intact.

I administered the Memory Impairment Screen, the Clock Drawing Test, and the Mini-Mental State Exam—all of which were normal. She passed all the items on the Direct Assessment of Functional Status, and she also scored in the competent range on the Hopkins Competency Assessment Test. More thorough testing using the Dementia Rating Scale and the Wechsler Memory Scale, however, revealed severely impaired short-term memory. But her mood assessment showed no significant signs of depression, and facility staff corroborated this. As a result, I diagnosed her with alcohol-induced memory problems (not with dementia, because while she had memory problems, she had no other thinking deficits), and here's what I recommended to the court:

1. Recognizing the importance of prudently monitoring Ms. Daniels's medical, cognitive, and psychiatric conditions and with all due respect to the need to protect Ms. Daniels from harm, it appears that at this time regarding her medical, financial, and living choices that Ms. Daniels is cognitively capable of making her own decisions.

2. However, given her high potential for alcohol relapse and her denial of having problems with alcohol, it is recommended that Ms. Daniels enter a residential alcohol treatment program. There, Ms. Daniels could be monitored and her past problems with alcohol more fully assessed, confronted, and treated.

3. If Ms. Daniels successfully completes a residential alcohol treatment program to the satisfaction of the program staff, she should be placed for at least six months in a supervised aftercare setting where her potential for relapse, cognitive status, functional capabilities, and medical concerns could be monitored. Twelve-step programming like Alcoholics Anonymous is also recommended.

4. If she remains relapse-free, her cognitive and psychiatric conditions should be reevaluated. If no significant changes to her cognitive and psychiatric conditions have occurred, and with continued close supervision, Ms. Daniels should be allowed to choose where and how she would like to live.

Thus far, I've talked about the key characteristics of Alzheimer's, other dementias, delirium, the natural process of aging, and the distinctions among them. I have also described some of the assessment tools available to measure the illness and its progression as well as concepts and processes involved in assessing thinking capacity. In the next two chapters, I will be discussing the insidious issues of depression and other serious mental health issues so commonly experienced by people with Alzheimer's.

Caretakers and the people they serve are all in a process of learning. They should not be afraid to acknowledge what they don't know. To admit what you don't know takes courage, because it leaves your vulnerabilities open and exposed. To this, however, I would say *face your fears anyway,* because to do this allows just the right teachers to enter your life. And with that, your uncertainty can diminish. It's a brave thing for an Alzheimer's sufferer or their caretaker to acknowledge what they don't know. But doing so anyway is the very thing that allows the help we all need, at times, to emerge.

Part 3

# Disturbances in Mood and Perception

# 10

# Geriatric Depression and Alzheimer's

"The heart is like a garden. It can grow
compassion or fear, resentment or love.
What seeds will you plant there?"

"Why am I still here?" "When my husband died I lost everything!" "I just feel tired all the time." "I worry that something bad might happen." These are statements commonly made by elderly people who are depressed, and although they are not always aware of it, people with Alzheimer's have good reason to be depressed.

There is general agreement that depression and other drastic changes in mood are the most common mental health problems in the elderly. According to the latest surgeon general's report, as many as 20 percent of older adults in the general population and up to 37 percent of residents in nursing homes and other primary care settings suffer from some kind of depression.[1] Risk factors for depression in the elderly include widowhood, physical illness, heavy alcohol consumption, financial problems, and a family history of mood problems.[2] How much stress we face does not, in and of itself, however, determine whether we feel depressed—what is equally important is how well we cope with the stress we have.

As we have seen, Alzheimer's wreaks havoc on a person's ability to think and act. It leaves confusion and devastation in its wake, and although many people with Alzheimer's are not clinically depressed, many are. Depression is most commonly seen in the earlier stages of the illness.[3] Although the prevalence of depression in the general population declines over the life span, as we get older, the severity of symptoms for those who are depressed increases. If people first become depressed after age 60, apathy and cognitive dysfunction become more prominent parts of their symptom profile. This may be due to a relationship between vascular disease and a particular type of depression that only first appears in later life. Studies have shown that people who have their first depressive episode late in life commonly show irregular, scalloped-edged bright spots on their magnetic resonance imaging (MRI) scans. These bright spots are found predominantly in the frontal lobe and are signs of vascular disease. This type of depression is referred to as *subcortical ischemic vascular depression* and at even modest severities is considered a significant risk factor for developing dementia.[4]

Typically, though, the most common symptoms of depression across the life span are

- depressed mood most of the day nearly every day;
- markedly diminished interest or pleasure in most activities;
- significant and unintentional weight gain or loss (greater than 5 percent);
- too much or too little sleep;
- diminished ability to think, concentrate, or make decisions;
- restlessness or, at the other extreme, slowing down of speech or movements;
- fatigue or a loss of energy nearly every day;
- feelings of worthlessness, guilt, or low self-esteem; and
- recurrent thoughts of death or suicide.[5]

Just how severe these symptoms are and how many of them a person experiences can vary. The more severe the symptoms and the more symptoms that are present, the more serious the depression. Real concern should arise if the symptoms last for two weeks or longer.

When people think of depression, the subjective feeling of sadness, hopelessness, or worthlessness usually comes to mind, but clinical depression in the elderly can take disguised forms, and people who have Alzheimer's will often exhibit atypical forms of depression. For example, *anhedonia* (the loss of enjoyment of life) is a very common symptom of depression in the elderly, as are repetitive health complaints, agitation, irritability, and worry. One of my nursing home patients put it well when she told me, "I've lost my joy. It's a lonely place here without my son. It's a scary thing to be here and not go home. It's hard to calm myself down. I feel afraid."

One of the tools clinicians use to measure depression in the elderly is called the Geriatric Depression Scale, and a short form of it is shown in figure 10a.[6] Easy and quick to administer, the Geriatric Depression Scale addresses issues of emptiness, boredom, fear, helplessness, isolation, worthlessness, fatigue, and overall life dissatisfaction. When the person is aware and fully able to report his feelings and perceptions, this particular measurement instrument can be useful, and as I described earlier, about two-thirds of Alzheimer's sufferers are either aware or partially aware of their illness.

**Figure 10a.** The Geriatric Depression Scale—Short Form

Ask the person to choose the best answer ("Yes" or "No") to each of the fifteen questions below. The questions should be framed in terms of how the person has felt over the last week.

| | | |
|---|---|---|
| 1. | Are you basically satisfied with your life? | Y <u>N</u> |
| 2. | Have you dropped many of your activities and interests? | <u>Y</u> N |
| 3. | Do you feel that your life is empty? | <u>Y</u> N |
| 4. | Do you often get bored? | <u>Y</u> N |
| 5. | Are you in good spirits most of the time? | Y <u>N</u> |
| 6. | Are you afraid that something bad is going to happen to you? | <u>Y</u> N |
| 7. | Do you feel happy most of the time? | Y <u>N</u> |
| 8. | Do you often feel helpless? | Y <u>N</u> |
| 9. | Do you prefer to stay at home rather than going out and doing new things? | <u>Y</u> N |
| 10. | Do you feel you have more problems with your memory than most people? | <u>Y</u> N |
| 11. | Do you think it is wonderful to be alive now? | Y <u>N</u> |
| 12. | Do you feel pretty worthless the way you are now? | <u>Y</u> N |
| 13. | Do you feel full of energy? | Y <u>N</u> |
| 14. | Do you feel that your situation is hopeless? | <u>Y</u> N |
| 15. | Do you think that most people are better off than you? | <u>Y</u> N |

Underlined responses are worth one point each. A score of 5 or greater indicates probable depression.

*From Sheikh and Yesavage (1988). Used with permission.*

Just as depression can be caused by vascular disease, research is beginning to show that depression in Alzheimer's may also be caused by the disease itself. For example, studies have documented that compared to non-depressed Alzheimer's patients, depressed Alzheimer's patients have more neuronal loss in brain centers controlling the generation of serotonin and norepinephrine—key neurotransmitters that are deficient in people who are depressed. There is also new evidence indicating that people who are not aware they have Alzheimer's are just as likely to be depressed as those who are.[7] As the person becomes less reliable in providing accurate information about himself, the observations of others become more important. In these cases, the Cornell Scale for Depression in Dementia is a useful assessment tool, and a complete list of items comprising this scale is included in appendix D, figure 5.[8] When a person with Alzheimer's cannot reliably report how he feels, this instrument allows the clinician to deduce from the behavioral observations of others the presence and severity of their depression.

When symptoms of depression become severe, the threat of suicide must be considered. Suicide completion rates for people over 65 are higher than for any other age group. This is especially true for males over 85.[9] Other factors that increase the likelihood of suicide are a history of substance abuse, recent losses, prior suicide attempts, and the presence of other psychiatric conditions. When family members or friends begin to hear things like, "People would be better off without me," "What's the use of living," "I just can't go on like this," "I've run out of hope," "I wish I wouldn't wake up tomorrow," "Why should I keep on living," or when the person begins to have a morbid preoccupation with death, or begins collecting pills, or withdrawing excessively, or not eating, the possibility of suicide must be considered. At this point, certain key questions must be addressed:

◆ How lethal are the person's thoughts and intentions?
◆ Does the person have the means to do it?
◆ Does he have a plan to do it?
◆ Does he intend to do it?

Clinicians have found that the best way to assess for suicide is just to ask the person directly. Despite uncomfortable feelings being stirred to the surface—usually more so for a friend or relative who may be asking—most of the time, the person is actually relieved to have someone he can talk to about it. It's a huge burden contemplating suicide, especially facing it alone. If you feel someone may be at risk for suicide, here are some questions you can use to broach the subject with him. They are listed in order of escalating intensity:

"What do you think about the future?"
"Do you feel like life may not be worth living?"
"Have you had thoughts of your life ending?"
"Have you thought about suicide?"
"When you think of suicide, what goes through your mind?"
"How often have you thought about suicide?"
"What would you use to end your life?"
"Do you have the means to do it—that is, do you have the weapon, the pills?"
"Have you thought of a plan on how you would end your life—that is, the time or place?"
"Are you serious about going through with it?"

If the answer to any of these questions is "Yes," then an immediate consultation with a physician, psychologist, or other appropriately trained clinician is advised. If appropriate, a sound suicide prevention plan should then be set up.

Just as symptoms similar to Alzheimer's are sometimes better explained by another medical condition, symptoms typical of depression, such as poor sleep, poor appetite, or poor concentration, may be better explained by an illness or disorder other than depression. For example, concentration problems or a depressed mood are also symptoms of anemia or hypothyroidism and these would first need to be ruled out before concluding it was clinical depression.

Diagnostic issues regarding Alzheimer's can become quite complicated because problems with memory (which might first appear to implicate Alzheimer's) can also be caused by concentration problems inherent in many types of depression. What might appear to be Alzheimer's but turns out to be clinical depression used to be called *pseudodementia* and is now referred to as *dementia syndrome of depression*. Both diagnoses—Alzheimer's and dementia syndrome of depression—frequently involve problems in concentration, comprehension, memory, mood swings, sadness, apathy, and sleep disturbance.[10] In both depression and Alzheimer's, a person may be unable to properly copy simple drawings, manipulate colored blocks, or arrange pictures in sequence to tell a story.[11]

One of the differences, however, between depression and Alzheimer's is that in depression, results from memory tests are often close to normal, whereas with Alzheimer's they are not. The more problems there are with memory and language, however, the more likely the presence of Alzheimer's and the less likely that it's simply depression. People with depression tend to report specific symptoms. With Alzheimer's, the complaints are usually quite vague. With depression, people will likely minimize their accomplishments, but with Alzheimer's they usually don't. With people who are depressed, memory prompting is helpful to stimulate recall, but with Alzheimer's it often isn't. A depressed person may not put forth much effort in the testing process, but people with Alzheimer's will usually make a good effort to do what's asked of them.[12] For more information on the difference between Alzheimer's and dementia syndrome of depression, take a look at appendix D, table 4.

Living with depression and living with someone who is depressed have their similarities. To help someone who is depressed, you need to understand, identify, and be able to sit with their suffering, especially when the person is denying it. This is not easy, but your compassion feeds their courage, your respect ministers their fear, and your bond with them soothes their pain. As a caregiver or as a loved one of someone who suffers from Alzheimer's, this is a garden worth tending.

# 11

## I Know She Has Alzheimer's, But Why Is She Acting Like This? Recognizing Psychotic Symptoms in Alzheimer's

> "Let yourself be open and life will be easier. A spoon of salt in a glass of water makes the water undrinkable. A spoon of salt in a lake is almost unnoticed."

As Alzheimer's disease strips away the ability to think clearly, it also diminishes the ability to cope with stress. When this happens, more serious mental health issues can arise. For example, because financial transactions are recalled more poorly, some people with Alzheimer's begin to believe that someone else is spending their money. For anyone, the prospect of this would be terrifying, but for people with Alzheimer's, it's especially true. If their understandable fear is not balanced by reasonable explanations, fleeting fear can turn into panic, and momentary suspiciousness into paranoia. When perceptions cannot be explained with rational reasoning and common sense, the Alzheimer's sufferer will resort to irrational means. Although depression and anxiety are more prevalent earlier on in the progression of the disease, excessively aggressive behavior, psychotic symptoms, and other irrational processes are more often exhibited in later stages of the illness.[1] Estimates are that over 65 percent of all the residents in nursing homes suffer from some type of psychiatric disorder.[2]

Florence was 91. Adult Protective Services entered her life because she could no longer care for herself. She had no known family, so the court decided to place her in a local nursing home. Fiercely independent and never married, for the first time in over 70 years, Florence was being asked to share a room with someone else. This was a huge adjustment for her. She was frightened when others entered her room, and she could not quite make sense that people in her room were nursing home staff or relatives of her roommate. The white tennis shoes in which she felt so comfortable were soiled one day by food she had spilled, and with her permission the laundry service was cleaning them. When she could not find her shoes, she swore that "the intruders stole them." Her beliefs intensified, and Florence began to feel she was being persecuted.

When the Alzheimer's sufferer holds strong beliefs that are persistent and yet irrational, they are called *delusions*.[3] For Florence, these delusions were paranoid or persecutory delusions—the only way she felt she could make sense of her surroundings was to believe that intruders were involved. For people who suffer from Alzheimer's, delusions can take a variety of forms. For example, in her spouse's absence, the Alzheimer's sufferer might begin jealously assuming that her spouse was being unfaithful, had abandoned her, or was plotting against her. A client I had seen for an evaluation at my outpatient practice felt she was being threatened by intruders whom she believed were entering her apartment. It turned out that she was just overhearing the actual voices of others in an adjoining apartment. She reported to me, "The building owner is behind it. He disguises himself, and he has talked to my doctor." She went on to say, "An electrician wired up my apartment, so he could eavesdrop on me." (I had later learned she was referring to a real person, an electrician, whom she had known years before my interview with her.) Patients will often develop elaborative rationale to explain their beliefs. Research suggests that paranoid delusions are quite common in Alzheimer's and are three times more likely to occur in people who are deaf than in the population at large.[4]

Delusions can also be grandiose (when a person holds an inflated sense of her own worth, own power, or own knowledge), erotic (when the belief is held that someone, usually of higher status, is in love with her), or somatic (the belief that parts of her body are misshapen, malfunctioning, or are infected or infested). Another form of delusion, called a referential delusion or *idea of reference,* refers to a psychotic condition where a person believes that random or unrelated gestures, comments, song lyrics, or newspaper headlines are specifically directed at her. One of my elderly patients with Alzheimer's believed that people on television were talking to her. When asked why she felt that way she replied, "They tell me 'Don't touch that dial!'" What leads a person to form one type of delusion or another is not quite clear but may depend on how much they may have been inclined to be jealous, suspicious, hypocondriacal, or grandiose prior to the onset of the illness. Delusions seem to be a function of biochemical changes caused by the disease combined with active thinking processes used by the person to explain her distorted perceptions.

Hallucinations are another form of psychosis in Alzheimer's.[5] Hallucinations are disturbances in sensory perceptions—that is, tricks the mind plays on us that tell us we are hearing, seeing, smelling, tasting, or feeling things that aren't there. While auditory hallucinations (e.g., hearing voices) are more common in the general population, visual hallucinations (seeing things that aren't there) are more common in Alzheimer's.[6] These distorted perceptions can take the form of people, animals, insects, or structural changes in one's surroundings. One of my nursing home patients remarked to me, "I don't go out of my room, because it is not safe. I can see the basement through the floor." This particular nursing home had no basement. Auditory hallucinations are not uncommon in Alzheimer's, though, and are perceived as voices that take on a life of their own. Although sometimes friendly, when malevolent, auditory hallucinations can be perceived as demanding or even commanding. When distortions of thought involve fears of being harmed by others, the person may come to believe that aggression is justified for self-defense.

Understanding psychotic symptoms in the Alzheimer's sufferer becomes a little more complicated by the fact that hallucinations and delusions can also be caused by severe depression, mania, schizophrenia, or by any number of medical problems such as hypothyroidism or hyperthyroidism, Addison's disease, Cushing's disease, Parkinson's disease, stroke, and other neurological disorders. Estimates are that 30–40 percent of depressed Alzheimer's patients have psychotic symptoms. Whatever the cause, stress makes psychotic symptoms worse.

What is not a form of hallucination or a symptom of psychosis, but is considered to be the most common form of perceptual disturbance in Alzheimer's, is what's called an *illusion.*[7] In an illusion, people do not manufacture a voice or vision but misinterpret actual sights or sounds from their surroundings. Quite common is when Alzheimer's sufferers hear others talking through an open window or doorway and believe they hear their own names being called or perceive that others are in their room talking to them. People with Alzheimer's will often misinterpret a shadow in the room to be another person. This is not psychosis. To illustrate this further, one of my patients reported to me that she was being threatened by a man and a woman who entered her apartment without her permission. As she stated it, "They talk to me through the heating vent but I can't see them." This patient actually lived in an old building where the voices of others carried though the heating vents. She was not hallucinating or hearing imaginary voices. She was, however, misinterpreting the very real voices of others that she was actually hearing. People with Alzheimer's are constantly trying to make sense of and sort out issues in their internal and external worlds. The troubling consequence of this is that they can overinterpret what they see and hear. This type of misinterpretation, however, is not considered in and of itself a form of psychosis.

Marge was a ten-year resident of her nursing home. Legally blind, she had been institutionalized with paranoid schizophrenia for much of her adult life. When her mobility began to fail and her dementia and other medical conditions became too much for her family caretakers to manage, she was admitted to a skilled nursing facility. In order to address issues of depression and to help her manage her psychotic symptoms, for almost three years I saw Marge for weekly supportive counseling. Like many people with chronic schizophrenia, she was a bit of an isolationist. My constancy in her life allowed her to quell many of her paranoid thoughts, and she made remarkable progress. For the first time in many years, she was successfully managing most of her troubling and long-standing psychotic symptoms. Her solitary lifestyle, however, unintentionally reinforced her chronic feelings of loneliness. As does happen sometimes, changes in my own life eventually forced me to turn her psychological care over to another clinician, and we spent two months planning for the transfer.

Marge had always maintained certain delusional beliefs—some malevolent, others benign. In the waning weeks before my departure, Marge began to voice her sadness with our impending termination, and this was clinically therapeutic for her. She also began to tell me about the new and pleasant experience she was having on "the boat," so asked her about it.

*Marge:* I will miss you.

*Dr. Kraus:* Yes. It's sad that our therapy together is going to end. You have made great progress, and I am proud of you. I know you will continue your good work with Dr. Hamilton. You had mentioned to me about a boat. Can you tell me more about it?

*Marge:* Oh, yes! We travel around.

*Dr. Kraus:* Do you, now! Where have you been?

*Marge:* We're going to France.

*Dr. Kraus:* Really! How nice! It sounds like a cruise ship.

*Marge:* Not really. [whispering] It's a submarine, but you can't tell anyone.

*Dr. Kraus:* How come?

*Marge:* They might throw me off.

*Dr. Kraus:* I see. What's it like for you traveling to all these places?

*Marge:* There's a group of us . . . my roommate . . . and a few more . . . and Nancy [one of her nursing assistants] . . . I like it.

*Dr. Kraus:* That's terrific. It sounds like you're seeing that while you are sad our therapy is ending, you also see that you will have some good friends here with you after I am gone.

*Marge:* [Smiling and in a very calm and self-assured voice] Yes, I will.

Many of the elderly people I have evaluated for Alzheimer's are savers—they save old newspapers, paper bags, almost anything. When memory fails, people with Alzheimer's become more unsure of themselves. Hanging on to things can provide a sense of security, and letting go of things can feel like a big risk. After all, they might need it! One of my Alzheimer's patients had saved so much of her own trash that she had actually been walking around her home not on her flooring but on debris built up for years. Alzheimer's creates other serious mental health issues. Figure 11a presents a summary of the ones we've discussed.

Just how persistent the symptoms are and to what extent people can accept the truth even when it contradicts their own perceptions or beliefs are two primary factors determining how big a problem these symptoms will create for themselves or others. The more rigid the person's beliefs or perceptions, the more stressful the symptoms will be. If the person's beliefs and perceptions are pliant, she can reinterpret them from a less agitating and distressing perspective.

It's a difficult thing to provide care to someone with Alzheimer's. It takes skill and patience. We often become impatient when we feel out of balance, when we struggle with our capability to help others, when our expectations get too high and do not appropriately match the situation in which we find ourselves.

Balance is restored, however, when we can begin to accept our helplessness, self-nurture our feelings of rejection, or self-soothe our sense of despair. When we do this we open ourselves to the whole of our own lives and to the lives of the people for whom we provide care.

---

**Figure 11a.** More Serious Mental Health Issues of People with Alzheimer's

**Delusions**
- ◆ Paranoid or persecutory delusions
- ◆ Delusions of jealousy
- ◆ Grandiose delusions
- ◆ Delusions of abandonment
- ◆ Delusions that someone on TV was talking to them

**Hallucinations**
- ◆ Visual hallucinations—seeing things that aren't there (the most common in Alzheimer's)
- ◆ Auditory hallucinations—hearing things that aren't there (not uncommon)
- ◆ Olfactory hallucinations—smelling things that aren't there (less common)
- ◆ Tactile hallucinations—feeling things on or inside our skin that aren't there (less common)

**Illusions**
- ◆ Hearing others talking outside the room and believing they were talking to us when they were not
- ◆ The belief that in a dark room a chair was actually a person
- ◆ The perception that characters on TV were really in the room

**Behavioral Disturbances**
- ◆ Wandering
- ◆ Verbal outbursts
- ◆ Agitation and restlessness
- ◆ Sundowning
- ◆ Threats of violence or suicide

Part 4

# Medical and Psychological Treatment Approaches

# 12

# Treatment of Alzheimer's with Medicines

> "I am happy today. I realize this was not yet a posthumous tale."[1]

Treating Alzheimer's dementia is indeed a complex undertaking. The illness affects a person medically, psychologically, socially, and spiritually. Therefore, in order to optimally impact the person's emotional and intellectual life, the illness must be treated using a variety of approaches. More will be discussed in the next two chapters on psychological and social treatment interventions for Alzheimer's, but for now, I would like to address the brain chemistry of Alzheimer's and how the illness can be treated with medicines.

The historical treatment of Alzheimer's with medicines is a story with good news and bad news. Let's get the bad news out of the way first. There are two principal classifications of medicines that are used today to treat Alzheimer's: cholinesterase inhibitors and glutamate inhibitors. In a minute, I will talk about these classes of drug treatments and how they can help, but you should know that these drugs are often only imperceptibly effective. Researchers at the forefront of the fight against Alzheimer's have said:

Treatment of dementia with cholinesterase inhibitors or memantine can result in statistically significant, but clinically marginal improvement in measures of cognition and global assessment of dementia.[2]

This means that researchers can measure small differences using statistical comparisons of treatment and no-treatment groups, but the person who is afflicted with Alzheimer's or other people in their life may not be able to see any real differences in their memory or their behavior. These medicines are designed to slow the progression of the disease, but it is unclear how well they do this. This was primarily the reason why over the last ten years the promise of a cure for Alzheimer's has faded. Between 2002 and 2012, 99 percent of drug research failed to produce the desired effects in treating Alzheimer's, and the research was either halted or stopped. Some of the more highly touted drugs that once held promise included Alzhemed (a beta amyloid aggregation inhibitor), Bapineuzumab (a passive vaccine), Flurizan (an anti-inflammatory), Dimibon (a Russian antihistamine at one time believed to effect Alzheimer's), and Gammagard (an immune globulin intravenous therapy)—all of which failed to produce the intended results.

And yet there have been flickers of research that kept our hopes alive, and they will be the focus of this chapter—the current and newest medical treatment ideas that are on the scientific horizon. More is being learned about the illness all the time, and newer and more novel approaches are continually being undertaken to understand this mysterious illness. So, let's first begin with what's currently available to treat Alzheimer's and go from there. I am going to talk about cholinesterase inhibitors, glutamate inhibitors, secretase inhibitors, biomarkers, vaccines, and many other topics related to treating Alzheimer's. I will also talk about medications used to treat other psychiatric symptoms that commonly accompany the illness.

## Cholinesterase Inhibitors

To date, the greatest amount of medical research has been directed toward developing cholinesterase inhibitors. As I discussed in chapters 1 and 4, acetylcholine, central to memory and learning, has been thought to play a pivotal role in the development and spread of Alzheimer's. Just how much of this chemical is available in our brain appears to be related to the onset of the disease—that is, people with Alzheimer's seem to have less acetylcholine than people who don't. How this chemical is manufactured is a complex biochemical process, but in its simplest form, it's illustrated in figure 12a.[3]

**Figure 12a.** How Acetylcholine Gets Manufactured in the Brain

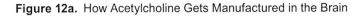

Choline Acetyltransferase

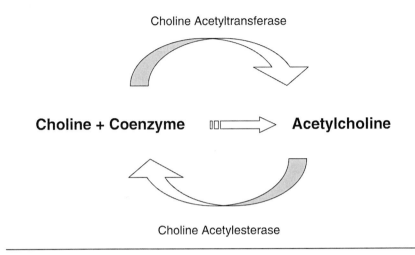

**Choline + Coenzyme** ▯▯▭⟹ **Acetylcholine**

Choline Acetylesterase

Acetylcholine is really comprised of two chemicals: choline and a coenzyme. Choline is an "essential nutrient" in that the body cannot produce it on its own and thus needs to acquire it from healthy foods. An enzyme is like a chemical catalyst that causes biochemical transformations, and a coenzyme is a substance that is like a vitamin that works with an enzyme to facilitate its activity. When we learn and remember things, acetylcholine continuously and repeatedly breaks into its component parts and then puts itself back together again. It breaks apart to do its work, and then restores itself to start the process all over again. This is a complicated biochemical undertaking, but the important thing to know about it is that the level of acetylcholine in the brain of the person with Alzheimer's is too low. Too little acetylcholine interferes with the proper storage and retrieval of learned material.

Also shown in figure 12a are two other important chemicals involved in the acetylcholine production process: (1) choline acetylesterase, which helps break acetylcholine apart; and (2) choline acetyltransferase, which helps put it back together again. When these two chemicals don't work as they should or are unavailable in sufficient quantity to do what work is needed, the whole process bogs down, the transformations do not proceed the way they need to, and the result is that memory and learning abilities decline. This is the central idea behind the cholinergic hypothesis: there is too little acetylcholine available in the brain (principally because there is too much choline acetylesterase—the chemical that breaks acetylcholine apart). Researchers believe that if there was a medication that inhibited the level of choline acetylesterase, then more acetylcholine would be available for learning and memory. This has been the fundamental principle guiding much of the earlier pharmaceutical research on treatments for Alzheimer's. Simply put, one of the two most commonly prescribed medications in the fight against Alzheimer's was designed to lower the level of choline acetylesterase in the brain, and drugs in this class are called choline acetylesterase inhibitors (or cholinesterase inhibitors, for short). To date, there have been several effective cholinesterase inhibitors introduced, and these medications are listed in table 12a. These medications do not cure the disease and only slow its progression temporarily.

Approved by the Food and Drug Administration in 1996, donepezil (trade name, Aricept) was introduced. It is widely prescribed and has shown some clinical effectiveness in lessening the symptoms of Alzheimer's and temporarily slowing the rate of the progression of the illness. Interestingly, donepezil is made from the extracts of daffodils and snowdrops. Rivastigmine (trade name, Exelon) and galantamine (trade name, Reminyl/Razadyne) were introduced in 2000 and 2001/2005, respectively, and are frequently prescribed for Alzheimer's as well. The general conclusion from research is that the

**Table 12a.** Cholinesterase Inhibitors Currently Used to Treat Alzheimer's Disease

| Drug | Severity Approval Level | Common Side Effects |
|------|-------------------------|---------------------|
| Donepezil<br>Brand Name: Aricept<br>Introduced: 1996<br>Manufacturer: Eisai/Pfizer | All severities of the illness | Nausea, vomiting, diarrhea, trouble sleeping, muscle cramping |
| Rivastigmine<br>Brand Name: Exelon<br>Introduced: 2000<br>Manufacturer: Novartis | All severities of the illness | Nausea, vomiting, diarrhea, dizziness, indigestion, hallucinations |
| Galantamine<br>Old Brand Name: Reminyl<br>New Brand Name: Razadyne<br>Introduced: 2001/2005<br>Manufacturer: Janssen | Mild to moderate symptoms | Nausea, vomiting, diarrhea, loss of appetite, dizziness, head pain |

effectiveness of cholinesterase inhibitors do not differ significantly from each other, only in their side effect profile.[4]

Studies have shown that the cholinesterase inhibitors can delay the progression of Alzheimer's by about 18 to 24 months and delay mild cognitive impairment, which eventually converts to Alzheimer's, by about 6 months. Based on the person's overall medical picture, the treating physician will decide which drug is the most appropriate choice.

After the physician prescribes a medication, the patient is monitored for changes in mental status, activities of daily living, and any other changes in his general behavior. Current practice protocols for the administration of cholinesterase inhibitors recommend that the drug be continued for 6 to 12 months if effective. Effectiveness can mean a reduction in symptoms or stabilization of further deterioration. Based on any changes in symptom severity, the physician makes adjustments to the dosage as needed.[5] The effectiveness of cholinesterase inhibitors is temporary, though. Eventually the disease overpowers the medicine and advances unabated.

## Glutamate Inhibitors

Glutamate is like caffeine in the brain—it excites other processes and functions, and too little or too much of it is not good. One of the 20 most common amino acids in the body (which are formed by DNA chains), glutamate is a very important neurotransmitter in the brain, and scientists are discovering that it may play an essential role in learning and memory. Several drugs have been designed to address abnormal glutamate levels, and they are listed in table 12b. The first of these was memantine.

Manufactured in Germany by Merz Pharmaceuticals for some ten years, memantine has been marketed throughout the European Union by Lundbeck as Ebixa and by Merz Pharmaceuticals as Axura. Memantine is not a cholinesterase inhibitor but acts like a kind of guard against excessive amounts of glutamate. In 2003, Forest Laboratories was granted FDA approval to market memantine in the United States as Namenda. Initial studies showed that Namenda might delay the decline in ADLs. Memantine was designed to treat the more severe symptoms typical of the later stages of Alzheimer's, and it has been approved for this use. In 2005, however, the FDA rejected memantine's use for people with mild Alzheimer's symptoms. In 2014, the FDA approved Namzaric—which is a combination of donepezil and memantine and covers all severity levels of the illness—for public use. Too little as well as too much

**Table 12b.** Glutamate Inhibitors Currently Used to Treat Alzheimer's
Disease

| Drug | Severity Approval Level | Common Side Effects |
| --- | --- | --- |
| Memantine<br>Brand Name: Namenda<br>Introduced: 2003<br>Manufacturer: Forest Laboratories | Moderate to severe symptoms | Confusion, cough, diarrhea, dizziness, head pain, infrequent bowel movements |
| Donepezil + Memantine<br>Brand Name: Namzaric<br>Introduced: 2014<br>Manufacturer: Actavis | All severity levels | Trouble sleeping, cramping, diarrhea, nausea, vomiting, confusion, cough, infrequent bowel movements |

glutamate may impact the progression of Alzheimer's, but no glutamate ago-
nists are currently approved by the FDA.

## Hope for the Future

The breadth of contemporary research on Alzheimer's includes a variety of
old and new approaches: exploring secretase inhibitors, untangling the tau
protein, using vaccines, monitoring genetic biomarkers, managing diet and
exercise, reducing insulin resistance, reducing circulatory problems, and other
perspectives.

**Secretase Inhibitors.** In contrast to the cholinergic hypothesis, the amyloid hypothesis proposes that excessive and abnormal beta-amyloid—a toxic protein—
is the root cause of Alzheimer's. Although some of the most recent research has
shown that abnormal beta-amyloid might be a chemical by-product formed to
protect the cell from the illness and may not be the cause of the disease, it is
more commonly believed that by stopping the production of this toxic protein,
the symptoms of Alzheimer's can be better controlled. Two classes of drugs have
been under clinical investigation designed to do just this: the beta-secretase and
gamma-secretase inhibitors. Recall from chapter 4 that these substances cleave
or cut the ends of the amyloid precursor protein resulting in the production of
toxic beta-amyloid. Research on these drugs is still in an early stage.

Alzhemed was one of the failed attempts to produce an FDA-approved secretase inhibitor, but the approach used to create this medicine was an innovative one. Researchers still believe that amyloid plaques form because molecules of the beta-amyloid protein "stick" to one another. The idea persists that if beta-amyloid could lose its stickiness, it would be less likely to aggregate and form amyloid plaques, and researchers have not given up on this idea.[6]

**Vaccines.** Rather than treat Alzheimer's after it has already developed and spread, why not create a vaccine against it? Two strategies are currently being used to vaccinate against the production of beta-amyloid plaques: one approach tries to block their further development after they appear and the second tries to prevent them from developing in the first place. There are two ways researchers believe vaccines can be used to immunize the body against plaques—through passive and active immunization. Passive immunization provides the afflicted person with the antibodies needed to fight the plaques directly through infusions. In 2014, when thousands of people in West Africa were dying of the Ebola virus, doctors successfully gave those infected an antibody to fight off the illness. Passive immunization does not endure, though—its success depends on getting more antibodies to the person as they may need them. On the other hand, active approaches to immunization help the body develop the antibodies it needs on its own—that is, the vaccine helps strengthen the person's immune system so it can produce the antibodies it needs for itself. With Alzheimer's, it is believed that ApoE-4 may be involved in the production of enzymes that could get blocked by an immunizing agent.[7]

Intravenous immunoglobulin therapy (IVIg) has been around for some time and is an FDA approved treatment for immune disorders in children. It has also been used to treat multiple sclerosis, toxic shock syndrome, and other illnesses in adults. It turns out, though, that IVIg also contains antibodies that bind to beta-amyloid and may help clear its toxic derivatives from the brain. IVIg research for Alzheimer's is being pursued.[8] Treatment costs for IVIg therapy, however, are currently estimated to range from $5,000–$10,000 per month.

**Biomarkers.** Early detection and management of Alzheimer's has relied on advances in biological indicators or biomarkers. Much of the research on biomarkers for Alzheimer's has focused on cerebrospinal fluid. Standardized methods are being developed to measure the amount of beta-amyloid in spinal fluid, which may be able to predict the development of Alzheimer's up to 30 years before the symptoms of the disease manifest.[9]

In 2012, the FDA approved the first radioactive tracer—named florbetapir F 18—that attaches to toxic beta-amyloid, which then can be seen in a PET scan. In 2013 and 2014, the FDA approved two other molecular imaging agents in detecting Alzheimer's—flutemetamol and florbetaben. The difficulty in coming to accurate and useful conclusions about the presence of beta-amyloid plaques is that many people who have these plaques do not have impairments in thinking or memory.

**Anti-inflammatories.** Initially based on anecdotal evidence that rheumatoid arthritis patients were less likely to get Alzheimer's, anti-inflammatory drugs have been explored as a potential treatment option for the disease. Although steroids like Prednisone showed poor outcomes, initial research on non-steroidal anti-inflammatories (NSAIDs)—drugs like Aleve and Advil—showed some promise. Research on long-term use of NSAIDs, though, has identified serious gastrointestinal problems, such as bleeding ulcers and liver toxicity, and kidney problems.[10] The general consensus on the effectiveness of NSAIDs seems to be that NSAIDS do not effect the severity of symptoms in Alzheimer's.[11] In fact, some recent research suggests that anti-inflammatory processes may actually trigger the disease.[12]

**Antioxidants.** In addition to the newer pharmaceuticals, there has been a significant amount of discussion about the role of so-called alternative medicines in the prevention and treatment of Alzheimer's. Among the most frequently discussed of these potential remedies are the antioxidants, folic acid, hormone replacement therapy, and various botanical treatments.

By way of some background, antioxidants seem to be a major source of good health and longevity, because they help cells in the body produce energy. Produced in the body and also found in natural foods, vitamins, and other nutrients, antioxidants help protect cells from harm. Cells are damaged by what are called free radicals, produced in the body but also found in pollutants, smoke, and other toxic substances. The damage that free radicals bring about is believed to be the major cellular cause of aging. Antioxidants, on the other hand, are believed to keep cells from aging and protect them from Alzheimer's. Two primary and natural sources of antioxidants are vitamin C and vitamin E, which are found in apples, berries, carrots, citrus fruits, garlic, onions, and green leafy vegetables.[13] Some research has shown that vitamin E limits free radical production and promotes the growth of neurons exposed to beta-amyloid. Although studies have shown that vitamin E could delay the progression of Alzheimer's, the estimates are by only about six months. However, drinking fruit and vegetable juices more than three times per week might reduce the risk for getting Alzheimer's. Not all vitamin Es are alike, though. What we know as vitamin E comes from a family of naturally occurring compounds called tocopherols, some of which may actually lead to increased beta-amyloid levels, so further research is needed to sort this out.[14]

Selegiline, used in the treatment of Parkinson's disease, also has antioxidant properties similar to vitamin E and has been shown to delay the progression of Alzheimer's, but again, only by very modest amounts.[15] For Alzheimer's sufferers, falls and fainting, however, are two long-term side effects of taking vitamin E and selegiline.

**Omega-3.** We've all heard a lot about omega-3 fatty acids. Commonly found in salmon, tuna, herring, and sardines, omega-3 fatty acids are a natural anti-inflammatory precursor. In one study, residents of nursing homes were followed for seven years, and it was found that those who ate fish at least once a week had a substantially lower risk of Alzheimer's.[16] However, the body of research on the impact of omega-3 fatty acids on lowering the risk for Alzheimer's disease seems to suggest that there may be a modest but measurable benefit from eating fish but, at best, a negligible benefit from omega-3 supplements.[17]

**Folic Acid.** Folic acid is a B-complex vitamin ($B_9$) that is commonly found in oranges, strawberries, beans, and dark green leafy vegetables, but it turns out that it is relatively scarce in Alzheimer's sufferers. There is substantial scientific literature supporting the idea that maintaining adequate folic acid levels is essential for good health. There is also research supporting the notion that maintaining satisfactory levels of folic acid can reduce the risk of Alzheimer's singificantly.[18] Keep in mind, though, smoking is especially detrimental in reducing folic acid levels.

**Stem Cells.** A lot of discussion has been generated lately around stem cell research, and it is considered to be as promising as it is controversial. Stem cells are generic or unspecialized cells that can be converted to form any cell in the human body, including brain cells. Some scientists believe that stem cell research holds the key to curing a range of life threatening degenerative illnesses, including Alzheimer's. Others disagree. The controversy is centered on the source of the stem cells used for research and treatment. Most stem cells are procured from fertility clinics where couples donate their unneeded frozen embryos. Setting aside the moral and political issues surrounding this method of procurement, stem cells may also be available from adult human tissue. Recently, stem cell researchers have produced precursors to working brain cells from adult bone marrow stem cells[19] and from adult skin cells.[20] As a possible cure for Alzheimer's, though, this research has a long way to go.

**Hormone Replacement Therapy.** While it has been well known that women live longer than men and eventually would be more likely to develop Alzheimer's, the initial research found that controlling for age, there was no difference in the incidence of Alzheimer's in men and in women. However, the general consensus from more recent studies supports the idea that women more than men are at greater risk for Alzheimer's. The earliest theories proposed that Alzheimer's in women resulted from deficiencies in the hormone estrogen following menopause. Hormone replacement therapy (HRT) was initially believed to have beneficial effects on postmenopausal women with Alzheimer's, but newer research has demonstrated that HRT may only be effective when administered during a "critical period" earlier in life. Research has also found that HRT increases the risk of stroke. This has led the National Institute on Aging to recommend that hormone replacement therapy should not be prescribed for older women to maintain or improve cognitive functioning.[21]

Newer research has proposed a related but alternative hypothesis involving hormonal imbalances in the hypothalamus-pituitary-gonadal (HPG) axis—where estrogen, testosterone, and other key hormones in both men and women are controlled. One of these essential hormones, luteinizing hormone (LH), is likely to be three to four times the normal level in postmenopausal women and twice the normal level in post-andropausal men. LH also has been found to be particularly elevated in people with Alzheimer's. Researchers are proposing that any chemical compound that inhibits LH may be a potentially effective preventive treatment for Alzheimer's.[22]

**Ginkgo Biloba.** Research has shown that botanical treatments, like Ginkgo biloba, may also have positive effects on the illness. Ginkgo biloba is type of subtropical tree whose leaves may decrease decline in thinking abilities due to Alzheimer's. Studies of Ginkgo biloba have shown a small decrease in the rate of thinking decline (usually around 2–3 percent) but have also shown an increase in reported gastrointestinal problems.[23] There is also evidence that Ginkgo biloba (especially when taken with blood thinners used to combat heart disease) may dangerously reduce the blood's ability to clot. The most recent research on Ginkgo biloba shows, however, no clinical effect in reducing cognitive decline over placebo control groups.[24]

**Chelation Therapy.** I never would have imagined we have hydrogen peroxide ($H_2O_2$) in our brain. We do, though, and its concentration level is relatively high because brain tissue consumes a lot of oxygen. This is important to consider because there is growing evidence that hydrogen peroxide may interact with metal ions (what comprises iron and copper) and beta-amyloid in the development of Alzheimer's. Chelation therapy—a blood filtering process that can remove heavy metals from the body—is being examined as a way of inhibiting the production of these toxic metal-containing substances.[25]

**Type 3 Diabetes.** More and more is being discovered about the relationship between Alzheimer's and diabetes, to the point that some researchers liken Alzheimer's to a "Type 3 diabetes." A great deal is known about two types of diabetes: Type 1 diabetes, which is an autoimmune disorder and accounts for 5 percent of all the cases of diabetes, and Type 2 diabetes, which accounts for 95 percent of cases of diabetes. Type 2 diabetes is a disorder where the person becomes resistant to their own production of insulin. What's interesting about diabetes and Alzheimer's is that people with Type 2 diabetes are roughly twice as likely to develop Alzheimer's than those without diabetes, and researchers are taking a closer look at this area of study.[26]

**Diet.** A great deal of research has been devoted to dietary influences on the development of Alzheimer's, and these findings have been aggregated into a diet that has been shown to lower the risk for the illness. To date, the most effective diet found is the Mediterranean-DASH Intervention for Neurodegenerative Delay diet. The MIND diet incorporates ten brain-healthy foods and includes these two recommendations:

1. Base your diet on leafy green and other vegetables, nuts, berries, beans, whole grains, fish, poultry, olive oil, and wine.
2. Avoid red meats, butter and stick margarine, cheese, pastries and sweets, and fried or fast foods.

To maintain the diet, it is recommended that we eat three servings of whole grains, a salad, and one other vegetable, and drink one glass of wine daily.[27]

**Resveratrol.** Although the MIND diet calls for a daily glass of wine, research is unclear exactly what it is about wine that may be useful. Some research has shown that a naturally occurring chemical compound found in red grapes and dark chocolate—resveratrol—may help stabilize beta-amyloid levels. However, it should be noted that the amount of resveratrol used in these studies—about 2,000 mg. per day—is the equivalent of 400 bottles of red wine.[28] Research continues to explore this fascinating compound.

**Transcranial Direct-Current Stimulation.** Transcranial direct-current stimulation refers to the use of electrodes delivering very low currents to specific areas of the brain. This approach has been proposed as a possible treatment for major depression, schizophrenia, chronic pain, post-stroke aphasia, and more recently Alzheimer's. Although the research is in its earliest stages, the method is intended to increase or decrease neuronal activity, depending on the illness being treated. Some studies have shown that transcranial direct-current stimulation can improve thinking functioning in people with early-onset mild cognitive impairment (MCI).[29]

**Exercise.** Much has been written about the importance of exercise in healthy aging. It has also been shown to reduce the incidence of Alzheimer's. To take an example, one study followed 1,740 people over the age of 65 for six years and found that those who exercised three days per week or more had as much as a 40 percent risk reduction for acquiring Alzheimer's.[30]

**Curcumin.** Some very interesting research is being done on a common spice that many of us have on the shelf—it's curcumin, the active ingredient in the Indian spice turmeric. It turns out that curcumin has antioxidant characteristics, and it has anti-amyloid properties as well.[31]

**Marijuana.** Is marijuana the new gray matter? There is a growing body of research on the medicinal properties of pot—specifically THC (tetrahydrocannabinol), the active ingredient in marijuana. THC may lower beta-amyloid levels and enhance mitochondrial function in Alzheimer's. It also has been found that cannabinoid receptors—nerve receptors that are found in high density in the hippocampus—function poorer in people with Alzheimer's than in those who don't have the disease. Studies have also shown that rats infused with toxic beta-amyloid performed better on tests of mental functioning when they were injected with cannabinoids than when they were not.[32]

**DMFO.** Recent research on mice by a National Institute of Health funded Duke University study showed that a drug called difluoromethylornithine (DFMO) might inhibit the formation of sticky plaques. Here's what they found: in Alzheimer's, an immune cell called arginine that normally protects the brain seems to chew itself up in Alzheimer's. DFMO blocked this process in mice and prevented the formation of plaques.[33]

**Huperzine A.** Another area of research on Alzheimer's has focused on the promise of huperzine-A.[34] Huperzine-A is a moss extract commonly used in traditional Chinese medicine and is seems to have properties similar to FDA-approved cholinesterase inhibitors.

**Body Mass Index.** Older research examining the role of obesity and body mass index (BMI) on the prevalence of Alzheimer's found that people with a BMI of at least 30 (approximately 20 percent overweight) had a 74 percent greater likelihood of developing a degenerative brain disorder.[35] More recent research, however, has shown that the picture may be more complicated: high BMI in midlife appears to be a risk factor, but high BMI in late-life may be a protective factor.[36]

**Hippocampal Volume/Metabolism.** As we discussed earlier, the hippocampus plays an essential role in memory and learning. The most recent research has indicated that decreased hippocampal volume and decreases in the hippocampal metabolism of glucose might predict the illness years before Alzheimer's symptoms actually appear.[37]

**Blood Vessel Integrity.** Scientists are also learning that processes inside blood vessel walls may play a key role in the pathogenesis of the illness. Researchers at the University of Antwerp found that deterioration in the tiny vessel walls inside the brain seem to clog the vessel, trap the toxic beta-amyloid protein inside the brain, and prevent it from clearing across the blood-brain barrier. Other research is continuing to reveal the potential relationship between heart disease and Alzheimer's.[38]

**Gum disease.** Curiously, studies of identical twins have shown that gum disease may be a risk factor in Alzheimer's. Researchers have found that the twin who had severe periodontal disease prior to age 35 had a fivefold increase in their risk for Alzheimer's.[39]

**SQUID Magnotometry.** As I discussed earlier in the section on chelation therapy, heavy metals may play a role in the illness. More specifically, microscopic iron oxide crystals (called magnetite) may be involved in Alzheimer's. One novel method used to measure magnetite concentrations is a technique known as SQUID (superconducting quantum interference device) magnotometry. By examining magnetic fields and the dynamic electrochemical processes in the brain, SQUID technology can assess magnetite concentrations. With a treatment method called pulsed electromagnetic therapy, some researchers believe magnetite levels and the effects of Alzheimer's may be better controlled.[40]

## A Word about Cholesterol

As I have discussed, people with Alzheimer's frequently have other medical conditions, the most common of these being vascular problems like hypertension and coronary heart disease. Not only do these illnesses need to be treated for their own sake, but scientists are considering that Alzheimer's may itself be a type of vascular disorder that only later manifests in brain dysfunction.[41] It has been a replicated finding that diseases compromising the vascular system significantly increase the risk of Alzheimer's. For example, it's been found that African Americans with hypertension exhibit greater cognitive impairment and that the long-term use of hypertensives by African Americans may actually reduce their risk of cognitive decline.[42]

When I was diagnosed with coronary artery disease I had to lower my total cholesterol from 265 to what it is now—75. Knock on wood; this will help me fend off the illness. In the process, though, I've learned a few things about cholesterol. For one, did you know that 30 percent of the body's cholesterol is found in the brain? Interestingly, cholesterol exists in the brain in the form of the APO-E protein (discussed in chapter 4).

The biomolecular metabolism of cholesterol is an extremely complicated process, but there is one basic part of it that you might know more about than you think: lipids (like cholesterol and triglycerides) are fats that combine with apolipoproteins (like APO-E) to form lipoproteins. You have heard the word lipoproteins before, because when you get your cholesterol checked the doctor tells you the results of the cholesterol test in terms of your "good" cholesterol (the high density lipoproteins or HDLs) and your "bad" cholesterol (the low density lipoproteins or LDLs). Interestingly, human research has shown that excessive LDL cholesterol levels may accelerate the production of toxic beta-amyloid. Over the last ten years, the thinking has been that statins—medications like

Zocor, Crestor, and Lipitor—may be useful in preventing Alzheimer's disease. The latest research, however, does not bear this out. While it is believed that cholesterol plays a role in the development of Alzheimer's and that statins are useful in treating heart disease, at this time, statins are not recommended in the prevention of Alzheimer's.[43]

## Medicines That Address Other Mental Health Symptoms

About 50 percent of Alzheimer's patients have some kind of additional psychiatric disorder. The disease makes life infinitely more complicated and confusing, and it exaggerates any other thinking problems or emotional difficulties with which the person may have been struggling prior to the onset of the illness. To help an Alzheimer's sufferer cope with other mental health issues, a variety of medications are available to the physician.[44] Prescribing medications to the elderly can be very tricky business, however, because the elderly show an increased sensitivity to the therapeutic effects of medications and to their side effects.

Sleep is perhaps the most important activity in the life of the Alzheimer's sufferer, and it is essential that it get managed properly. When sleep problems arise it is vital to identify what may be causing them. For example, if daytime naps become excessive, poor sleep at night is more likely. In this situation, the first thing usually recommended is to reduce or avoid daytime naps. If this intervention is insufficient, a sleep medication may be needed. Medication would not likely be appropriate for a nursing home resident whose roommate was excessively noisy at night. Tending to the roommate's sleep problems or allowing the resident to switch rooms would be a less restrictive intervention than to introduce a sleep medicine. Sleep problems are also symptomatic of other disorders like anxiety or depression which, if properly treated, may result in improved sleep patterns. If the treating physician is going to prescribe a sleep medication, trazadone, Sonata, or Ambien are among the most commonly chosen for the elderly.

When symptoms of depression arise, reassurance, support from others, and counseling are considered the first lines of intervention. In fact, the clinical literature has shown that in remedying some types of depressive symptoms (e.g., apathy), medications may not be of much use. When counseling and support aren't enough, however, antidepressants like Prozac, Paxil, Zoloft, Celexa, or Lexapro are the first ones commonly tried. These are among the newest-generation antidepressants; they are very specific in targeting

the neurotransmitter serotonin and are in a class of drugs called selective serotonin reuptake inhibitors—or SSRIs, for short. Antidepressants like Wellbutrin,
Effexor, and Cymbalta—ones that target both the serotonin system and other
neurotransmitter systems involved in depression (like the norepinepherine and
dopamine systems)—are generally the next class of antidepressant that is tried.
Older antidepressants like amytriptaline, desipramine, nortriptyline (known as
tricyclics) are usually the last choice for today's elderly, because these drugs
tend to be more sedating, have other more pronounced side effects, and tend
to work against cholinesterase inhibitors.

In treating symptoms of depression, the generally accepted medication
protocol is to administer adequate dosing for four to eight weeks, and if there
is no response switch to or augment with another class of antidepressant (e.g.,
switching from an SSRI like Zoloft to a noradrenergic reuptake inhibitor like
Effexor). Psychotherapy should always be considered as an adjunctive therapy to
medications. If there was still no response the physician would then reconsider
the accuracy of the original diagnosis. Although still somewhat controversial, if
depressive symptoms do not respond to medication or psychotherapy, electroconvulsive therapy may be an option. Electroconvulsive therapy (ECT) is not
what it used to be. Today, ECT is delivered at mild levels, with very regimented
protocols, is targeted to very specific areas of the brain, and shows few of the
side effects it once did. Although rarely administered, it can be especially
useful for those patients with unrelenting agitation and active suicidality.[45]

When symptoms of prolonged and excessive euphoria or exaggerated
mood swings are observed—symptoms like prolonged irritability, extreme
talkativeness, fidgetiness, or racing thoughts—a psychiatric condition called
bipolar disorder (formally called manic depression) may be present. Symptoms
like these may also be mixed with symptoms of depression. To treat these types
of manic-depressive mood swings, a physician may prescribe a medicine like
Depakote, Tegretol, lithium or Lamictal. Lithium and Depakote require careful
and regular blood level monitoring.

Alzheimer's victims often are very anxious. The certainty of their world
as they have known it has been compromised in profound ways. When nonmedical means of helping the person cope with their escalating confusion and
self-doubt have been exhausted, anxiety medications may be appropriate. The
medication of choice today for general anxiety or even panic attacks is the SSRI.
When an SSRI is not chosen, physicians may prescribe a mild and slow-acting
anti-anxiety medication like Buspar. When anxiety is severe and accompanied
by agitation that might put the person or others at risk, a fast-acting anti-anxiety

medication like lorazepam (trade name, Ativan) is frequently prescribed. Ativan is very sedating, however, and when prescribed over extended periods of time can be addictive. Drugs like lorazepam and other benzodiazepines (like Valium or Xanax) can be troublesome for the Alzheimer's patient, because these drugs have been shown to further inhibit thinking abilities in Alzheimer's.

Years ago, psychotic symptoms were typically treated with such medications as Haldol, Thorazine, and Stelazine. Haldol is still commonly used in hospital emergency rooms, because it's powerful, fast-acting, and effective. Because of the long-term and often permanent side effects from these drugs, however, they are not commonly used today, particularly with the elderly. Because they have fewer side effects, the newer (or what's called atypical) antipsychotics, like Zyprexa, Risperdal, Abilify, and Seroquel, are more frequently prescribed for psychotic symptoms in the elderly. There is, however, a greater risk for stroke and death with the atypical antipsychotics.[46] In 2005, the FDA issued a public health warning advising for the judicious administration of these medications. Some medications may actually cause confusion, and it may be useful to consider "unprescibing" them. A list of these medications can be found in appendix D, table 5.

Medicines play a valuable role in the treatment of Alzheimer's and the problems with mood, thinking, and perception that often accompany it. For many elderly people, happiness may be so simple as a good night's sleep, but careful selection of medicines is critical and can make all the difference. After struggling with prolonged and agitated mood swings, one of my nursing home patients passionately told me, "I was in hell, and now I'm in heaven. I can think straight now." The effective use of medications not only can avert problems, but it can also transform the overall outlook of Alzheimer's sufferers by dramatically altering the quality of their lives as well as the lives of others around them for the better.

"Roses become compost; compost feeds the garden for the growth of new roses."[47] Our lives are but part of a larger cycle repeatedly acted out. Eventually, all things end only to begin anew in other forms. As caretakers, we can do only what we can for those with Alzheimer's. Know, though, that whatever is left that we cannot control will be transformed into what will evolve and eventually grow again.

# 13

## Changing the Person's Surroundings

"In one's family, respect and listening are the source of harmony."

Because Alzheimer's is a disorder with psychological and social implications, it cannot be treated by medicines alone. Although medicines can help reduce the progression of symptoms and take some of the edge off the stress of this illness, in treating psychiatric disorders medicines plus counseling is usually more effective than either intervention prescribed alone. Therefore, in the next two chapters, I will be examining a variety of nonmedical interventions designed to help caregivers better intervene into the inner and outer worlds of the Alzheimer's sufferer.

As memory and thinking decline, it becomes immensely difficult to adjust to life. The stress of losing your ability to think is overwhelming. Stress can come from too much stimulation or too little. Boredom and apathy can be just as dangerous to the Alzheimer's sufferer as fear and frustration. The source of that stress can come from real issues in the person's outer world or from the inner perceptions and mental constructions inside the person's mind. As figure 13a illustrates, added stress can produce increased confusion, which in turn can lead to greater stress, which can further exaggerate cognitive decline.

**Figure 13a.** The Vicious Cycle of Stress and Cognitive Decline

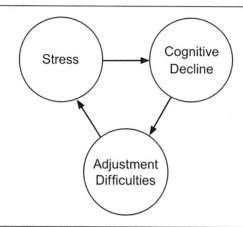

This is a vicious cycle, particularly for elderly people with Alzheimer's. Stress can be aggravated by the person's illness, triggered from their immediate physical surroundings, provoked by long-standing personality issues and coping styles, and intensified by other people in the person's interpersonal world. Although the caregiver is there to help, this person is unintentionally but frequently the source of some of this stress. These sources of stress are illustrated in figure 13b.

Treating stress in Alzheimer's by targeting problems in the immediate and surrounding situation is based on the idea of finding the right balance between too little and too much sensory stimulation. Stated somewhat differently, when our sense of sight or hearing or any of our other senses is assaulted, we react, even recoil. When the stereo is too loud we turn it down; when the room is too bright we lower the lighting; if it's too cold we turn up the heat. If we didn't, we'd be uncomfortable. We might find ourselves initially getting more irritable or frustrated, but when this happens we do something about it and get some relief. Common sense.

People with Alzheimer's, however, cannot think clearly enough to know what may be causing their irritation, anxiety, or confusion. They are not as aware that they are stressed. Even if they were, they may not know how to help themselves resolve it. But we can do something for them. We can help them by constructively managing their physical surroundings for them—that is, by making their surroundings more "Alzheimer's-friendly."[1] Following is a list of important environmental triggers that make it more difficult for people with Alzheimer's to adjust to the climate or atmosphere around them:

**Figure 13b.** Identifying the Causes of Distressing Behavior

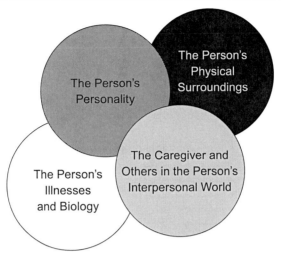

- ◆ Excessive noise
- ◆ Insufficient or excessive lighting
- ◆ Too little or too much activity
- ◆ Foul odors
- ◆ Too many changes too quickly
- ◆ Too many people around them
- ◆ Conversations with others that feel too complex, too argumentative or otherwise too intense

Consider how to eliminate or reduce these environmental triggers. Excessive noise has the potential of creating confusion and irritability, and in this case, the person's physical surroundings might be made more Alzheimer's-friendly by keeping things quiet and peaceful. To take another example, because nightfall can trigger sundowning, making lights brighter can help reduce sundowning as well as increase daytime activity. Increasing daytime activity, in and of itself, also can be very useful to better normalize nighttime sleep patterns.

John was one of my nursing home patients, and he was getting more agitated and irritable by the day. He also seemed more confused when his nurses entered his room. He reported feeling tired, and he was not getting very much sleep. The doctors ruled out infections, abnormal blood levels, and other medical issues that might account for the change in his condition. The staff assumed that John's symptoms were due to the progression of his Alzheimer's, and John himself could not explain his change in behavior. I consulted with the nighttime nursing staff, put John on 30-minute sleep checks, and developed a log to document what was being observed. Sure enough, John was restless at night and was only getting an hour or two of sleep at a stretch. What also was observed and documented, however, was that his new roommate was having a significant problem with sleep apnea and snoring, and the nursing staff noted that it was very loud. We asked John how he felt about his roommate's snoring. Reluctantly, John told us, "Well, I didn't want to say anything. After all, the guy just moved in here. But it keeps me awake." The nursing home moved his roommate down the hall and provided him treatment for his apnea. John got a new roommate who slept though the night, and as a result, so did John. In two days, John's irritability, confusion, and agitation began to diminish.

Keep in mind that whatever changes are made to a person's surroundings should be made slowly. For example, before John's roommate was moved we first talked with John (and his roommate). John agreed to try this intervention to see if it would be helpful, and we enrolled John in the process by letting him know what the nursing home's plan was and when it would be implemented.

To take another example, one of the most common behaviors in moderate to severe Alzheimer's is wandering and pacing. This is a real problem for any caregiver, and although redirecting the person into another activity or giving them medication to calm them are possible interventions, the newer thinking on wandering and pacing is to try to understand what the purpose of the behavior is—that is, before choosing an intervention, it is important to try to answer the following questions:

- Is the behavior aimless or is it goal-directed industriousness?
- Is it escapist?
- Is it akathisia-induced (a condition of inner restlessness caused by medication)?
- Is it a form of self-stimulation?
- Is it directed travel?
- Is it caused by the person's inability to find their way?
- Is it a role replay—that is, is the person enacting a prior role in life (e.g., acting out role behavior of a wife, a mother, a sibling, a worker)?
- Is the person searching for something?
- Is the behavior a form of exercise?
- Is the person in some discomfort?

Axs was a resident for many years in a nursing home in a quaint little village in the Midwest. One day when I came in to see her and to visit several other residents, I encountered several staff warning me, "Watch out for Axs today! She is in a sore mood!" As I entered Axs's room, I could see what they meant. Normally grateful to see me, Axs was grumpy and out of sorts. As I spoke with her about it, she really couldn't explain why she was so irritable, but as we talked I could see her wrestling with her garment and grumbling under her breath about how tight it was. Then I realized what was happening to her. I flagged down a nurse's aide and asked her to help Axs change into a comfier set of clothing. When I returned I could see she had calmed down, and by the time I left the session, she was back to her old self.

Researchers have developed some very useful rules (see figure 13c for a list of twelve) for optimizing the environment of older persons with thinking impairments—things like safeguarding their need for privacy and autonomy,

**Figure 13c.** Twelve Rules for Optimizing the Environment of Thinking-Impaired Older Adults

1. *Privacy*—a place to be alone with solitude
2. *Social Interaction*—opportunities to talk and share with others
3. *Control, Choice, and Autonomy*—the right to make (some) decisions for oneself and to control one's own life
4. *Orientation and Wayfinding*—a setting where it's easy to get around and know the way
5. *Safety and Security*—a place free from hazards and danger
6. *Accessibility and Functioning*—a place where there's easy access to doors, windows, and other features of the physical environment
7. *Stimulation and Challenge*—opportunities for stimulation, excitement, and challenge to combat boredom and apathy
8. *Sensory Aspects*—matching the lighting, sound, etc. to the needs of the older person
9. *Familiarity*—creating a setting where reminders of the person's past are considered and available
10. *Aesthetics and Appearance*—surroundings that are colorful, attractive, and provocative
11. *Personalization*—having a living space personalized by unique elements that express who the person is
12. *Adaptability*—an environment that is flexible and can adapt to the changing needs of the person

*Adapted from material taken from Regnier and Pynoos (1992). Used with permission.*

honoring their need for social interaction, creating an environment where reminders of the person's past are considered and available, and making the surroundings colorful and attractive.[2] Table 13b contains specific, nonmedical solutions to many commonly encountered problems in Alzheimer's. These suggestions are also designed around changing the afflicted person's surroundings. Take a look at these and see if any of them could be applied to your situation.[3]

**Table 13b.** How to Change the Surroundings for People with Alzheimer's

| Typical Problems | Recommended Strategies |
| --- | --- |
| Memory problems | Memory aides such as logs, notes, calendars, clocks |
| Losing things | Establish a place for things such as keys and wallet |
| Communication problems | Speak slowly and distinctly; reassure, smile, and touch |
| Attempts to "cover up" | Respect their denial; ensure emotional safety |
| Depression | Support; reassure; show empathy; seek professional help |
| Lack of motivation | Suggest activities and plans |
| Fear of losing control | Establish familiar and secure routines; encourage autonomy with simple tasks; praise accomplishments |
| Problems in judgment | Simplify decisions and tasks |
| Confusion and disorientation | Support; reassure; show empathy; provide structure |
| Safety concerns | Modify hazardous situations |
| Difficulties with ADLs | Simplify instructions |
| Changes in sexual behavior | Initiate intimate and affectionate exchanges; recognize impairments and limitations |
| Sleep disturbances | Discourage daytime naps; encourage exercise; consult the physician |
| Angry outbursts and agitation | Identify triggers; respond with calm reassurance; walk away; consult the physician |
| Problems in dressing | Offer help with choice of clothes; use simple directions; use special clothing (e.g., shoes with Velcro bands) |
| Decreased recognition of family and familiar places | Use links from the past; reassure; use repetition |

**Table 13b.** *(continued)*

| Typical Problems | Recommended Strategies |
| --- | --- |
| Eating problems | Create a slow mealtime pace; use finger foods or foods sized to be easily chewable |
| Incontinence | Use routine toileting; restrict fluids after evening; use an adult diaper; make sure you consult the physician |
| Falls | Eliminate safety hazards; provide adequate lighting; use a walker or cane; supervise ambulation; develop a plan to safely pick up the fallen person |

Adapted from Bozich and Housley (1985). Used with permission.

It's hard for family members to know just what to do with a loved one who's struggling with Alzheimer's. You may think you've tried everything. There is a Buddhist expression, though, that paradoxically advises, "Don't just do something, sit there!" Sometimes sitting and listening and taking in all that is around you can be challenging, but it also can provide a wealth of ideas on what to do. Sometimes just sitting with the Alzheimer's sufferer can be the best intervention of all. To understand and respect the disease, by just sitting with it and the person who has it, can be the very thing that can spawn creative solutions that just aren't unavailable to those who don't.

# 14

# Talking to People with Alzheimer's

"When someone loves you, the way they say your name is different. You know that your name is safe in their mouth."
—Billy, age 4[1]

The idea that we are all capable of lifelong learning is not new. Granted, some elderly folks may be more stubborn and set in their ways than others, but this can also be said about teenagers or Gen-Xers/Yers or baby boomers, or people from any age group. Being stubborn can also imply having mettle to take a stand and stick to it. Given the right circumstances, though, I believe that all people have the potential to make important changes in their lives. There is no more paramount an assumption than that when I talk to people with Alzheimer's. Despite their learning being slowed and their mental capabilities diminished, people with Alzheimer's (in all but the final stages of the illness) have the capability to find constructive ways to communicate their needs, to learn, and to grow in ways that go beyond words. The trick is learning their "language." What I plan to do in this chapter is to outline four basic strategies on how to talk to someone with Alzheimer's. Each approach presents a different perspective on how the listening and communication process might take shape and the impact it can have on the afflicted person and their family.

Before I do, though, I would like to offer one piece of advice over all others about how to talk to someone with Alzheimer's: *Use empathy generously.* Empathy is the ability to demonstrate understanding of what another person is thinking, what they might be feeling, what their words mean to you, what you think their words mean to them, and what they might be experiencing behind their words or actions. Empathy is the capacity to show another person that you know what it might be like to walk in their shoes. Empathy is at the bedrock of healthy relationships, and it sends the message, "Your feelings *matter* to me. *You* matter to me."

We show empathy when we set our own agenda aside just long enough to let the other person know they are not alone in their experience—that we understand them or that we want to understand them. It often involves being tenderhearted, compassionate, or sympathetic, but it can also involve identifying in a supportive way with another person's anger or resentment. This is especially important when dealing with someone about their disagreeable or aberrant behavior because while your intent may be benevolent, the other person's defenses will likely be heightened. And these elevated defenses may be unknowingly or unintentionally designed to prevent a dialogue with you, during which it might be discovered that your allegation about their aberrant behavior may be true. Confronting a person with Alzheimer's—however gently—is often seen by them as an intrusion, an invasion of their emotional space that will likely elicit their irritation. As a result, the response of the Alzheimer's patient is often to try to obliterate the accusation and often the messenger as well. This is where empathy rules. Here are a couple of examples.

> *Alzheimer's patient:* The nurse is abrupt with me. She treats me like a child. Before I retired, I had 50 men working under me! Who does she think she is?
> *Family member:* Who can blame you for feeling frustrated?

> *Alzheimer's patient:* I am terribly ill and can think of nothing but dying.
> *Family member:* How could you possibly think of anything else?[2]

The key to being empathic is learning how to set your frustrations aside just long enough to recognize that your loved one is hurting and that they are doing the very best they can to deal with their crippling illness. The typical

Alzheimer's patient lives with the idea that their mind is fading—some are aware of this and others are not. In either case, this is an incredibly frightening proposition. And understandably, they are not always willing to face it too squarely. So, for example, when you direct them to do something that they might not especially want to do or when they are upset, they likely will try to defend against seeing their illness in action. They won't want to look too directly at it. In this situation the key for you, the caregiver, is knowing and expecting that if you decide to direct them their tension level likely will rise. Here's what you do: anticipate their defensiveness; don't fight with it; prepare for it; flow with it; and use your empathy to welcome it as an opportunity to make a deeper connection with them.

## The Relationship Is Everything

A half-century ago, Harry Stack Sullivan changed the way we looked at emotional healing with a simple and profound idea.[3] At the time, the world of talk-therapy was steeped in three perspectives: (1) in Sigmund Freud's belief that unconscious aggressive and sexual impulses drove our behavior; (2) in Ivan Pavlov's notion that all behavior is acquired because it becomes conditioned to or associated with our natural reflexes; and (3) in B. F. Skinner's perspective that whatever we do, we do it strictly because we are trying to seek pleasure or avoid pain.[4] Sullivan proposed something different—that healing required an understanding of the person not in isolation from those around him but in the context of his relationships with others. What Sullivan was saying was that the character and climate of a person's interpersonal world profoundly influences the level of their felt distress.

Alzheimer's changes the way people relate to themselves and to others. When talking with someone with Alzheimer's it's important to listen to what the person may be saying about his past and present relationships with others and to pay attention to how he feels about himself. From this point of view, people with Alzheimer's need help with three principal issues: (1) how to adapt to the biggest transition of their lives—their changing health, getting older, and their changing family and work roles; (2) how to cope with the grief and loss that accompany the disease; and (3) how to manage their current interpersonal relationships with others.[5]

People with Alzheimer's go through immense life transitions—their roles in the family change, their views of themselves as mentally healthy people change, and their senses of their own longevity and mortality change. These are all extremely important issues that benefit from being discussed, examined, and worked through. If kept silent or hidden, the feelings underlying their transition often get acted out in a disguised form. Listening for references to the life changes with which Alzheimer's sufferers are struggling can be invaluable to them not only because it makes available a problem-solving process that may remedy the distress, but also because it brings a heightened sense of connectedness and bonding with you. When this happens, they are not alone and curiously, in that moment, neither are you.

Grief over family members that have passed on, sadness over their sense of lost usefulness, and loss of their former and more active pursuits that once gave them so much pleasure all make it more difficult for people with Alzheimer's to emotionally cope with the disease. Simply listening with supportive understanding and making meaningful emotional contact with Alzheimer's sufferers can bring them a sense of calm and solace. Although the person's memory for recent events may be lacking, long-term memory, especially for well-learned actions, events, and knowledge, is one of the last abilities to decline. In addition to empathically listening to their grief, what's often effective for people with Alzheimer's is to reminisce about the good times and people from their past, and I will be discussing more on how to do this in chapter 15. Talking with Alzheimer's sufferers is made easier by attentively listening for subtle references to the quality of significant relationships from their past. Those references are what can guide your responses, because the past is what Alzheimer's sufferers remember best. By helping them share something important and meaningful about their own lives, you bring into your here-and-now relationship with them the feelings of closeness they have experienced with others, and this makes the grieving process easier.

Desperately wanting to hold on to the joy from their past often creates avoidance of some of the troubled aspects of their current life, and people with Alzheimer's often have great difficulty managing their current relationships with others. Disagreements with family members and other care providers will often arise, and their sense of connectedness and support from others can feel lacking. Not only can they be more anxious, depressed, or impatient, the ability of Alzheimer's sufferers to use their own faculties to manage their emotional reaction to others is seriously impaired. Talking with Alzheimer's sufferers can take the form of supportively sitting with them while you help them revisit the strategies they have successfully used in the past to make their interpersonal world more fulfilling. As the effects of Alzheimer's take their toll, quietly listening to their current "people problems" without speaking can often be a big help, in and of itself.

Geraldine was one of my depressed nursing home patients with Alzheimer's and could not remember my name to save her life. I met with her every week for months, and at every session she had trouble recognizing me. "It's Dr. Sparky," I would say. The nursing home social worker who introduced me to each of my patients there liked telling them my nickname, and that's how everybody soon started knowing me. When she would hear this, Geraldine's brow and eyelids would rise ever so slightly. "I'm your psychologist," I would say. Barely recognizing me, I would prompt her recall with a verbal sketch of my role and why we were meeting. With this, you could begin to see her recognition building and she began feeling more at ease with me.

As a rule, Geraldine's mood was irritable; she had a cynical view of the world and she isolated herself excessively. Keeping to herself was a real problem for her, because she had begun to develop sores on her backside from lying in bed so much. When she wasn't in her bed she was lying in her recliner. Her sores were becoming so severe that the medical staff felt they would soon threaten her life. Despite forgetting who I was and what we had talked about the prior week, after a number of sessions together she began to learn at some level that she could trust me. One thing I enjoyed was her sarcasm, and she could see that. I encouraged her to socialize more with others, to give others a second chance; but it was not my expertise or even my words that made a difference—it was her trust in me that eventually allowed her to risk taking my suggestions to heart.

You see, underneath her rough exterior, Geraldine was really a sweetheart. As she allowed herself to experience trust in her relationship with me, she learned that she just might be able to better trust others as well. As she allowed others to know her, they began to see her sweetness, too, and as she socialized more, her depression began to lift—she spent less time in her bed and chair, and her sores began to heal.

Along with her physical healing, Geraldine experienced a significant emotional healing. Just how emotional healing occurs in therapy is still quite a mystery, but for Geraldine it seemed to occur at a level that went well beyond what she could articulate in words or what she could remember. In this sense, her Alzheimer's did not prevent her emotional recovery. Her learning seemed to take place not so much in her head but in her gut—as a consequence of how she felt about her relationship with me and later with others. Communication with her took place beyond words, beyond logic, beyond even conscious thought. And what happened to Geraldine is not unique.

I believe that this type of healing can occur because an emotional understanding is reached within Alzheimer's sufferers that has more to do with restored faith, with renewed hope, and with enhanced trust in the world, in themselves, and in their relationships with others than it has to do with cognitive functioning per se. Granted, the deterioration from Alzheimer's has a profound impact on these existential aspects of our being—the cognitive decline generates fear, anger, suspiciousness, loss, and any number of other difficult and challenging emotional experiences—but I believe that the disease process impairs emotional functioning on a cellular level only in the final stages of the illness. And that's why many people with Alzheimer's can be comforted and counseled, can feel the support you give them, and can reach a greater sense of peace with their illness. It's your empathy with their emotional experiences that eases their suffering. It's your empathy that cultivates their sense of joy in the life they are blessed to be living.

## Don't Take Their Words Too Seriously

It is universally acknowledged today that our behavior is often guided by motives about which we may only be dimly aware. This is what Sigmund Freud called the unconscious.[6] When repressed or denied feelings are brought into our awareness, we may not like them, and we may try to find ways to defend against experiencing them. We may deny that we are angry, hurt, or embarrassed even when those feelings are patently obvious to those around us. We may rationalize our poor decisions or project blame onto others for things for which we feel we are not responsible, even when we are. People with Alzheimer's are especially vulnerable to these kinds of reactions.[7]

As with any terminal illness, people with Alzheimer's attempt to construct a variety of strategies to cope with their disease. With or without deliberate intent, they may deny knowing or wanting to know that they have the illness. They may actively reject what losses their illness would predict or become angry with their illness or with others who may remind them of it. Other Alzheimer's sufferers may try to cope by attempting to preserve or reinstate what life they once had while actively ignoring what of life's beauty and splendor may still remain for them. Suffering from a terminal illness, others may try to revive a lifestyle they once knew but become anxiously concerned their body will not support their goals. Some Alzheimer's sufferers believe that self-destruction is the only way to cope with the disease. This can get played out through the excessive abuse of alcohol or drugs, by neglectfully shutting down their responsibility to care for themselves, by rejecting prescribed treatment regimens, by general recklessness, suicide, or by cutting themselves off from the goals, roles, and lifestyle with which they once identified and aspired to.[8]

Helping those with Alzheimer's get better in touch with the range of their own feelings and thoughts can be very helpful to them. From this perspective, the words they use are not as important as the feelings and meaning behind what they may be saying. Mirroring to them that you can grasp the deeper meaning of what they are trying to communicate can be invaluable to Alzheimer's sufferers and is what accurate empathy is all about. As Alzheimer's progresses, we've learned that a person's higher-order reasoning, his ability to think abstractly, and his insight into his own behavior diminishes. It stands to reason, then, that people with Alzheimer's have a more difficult time making sense of the motives behind their actions. They lose their capacity to answer the question, "Why did you do that?" Because of changes in their brain, their own actions and motives are made ever more difficult to understand and explain to others. Here's what I mean by this.

Grace was 89 and often wandered the nursing home hallways distressfully repeating the phrase, "I want to go home . . . I want to go home." The nursing staff tried to help her by reorienting her to her surroundings and would say with gentle supportiveness, "Grace, this is your home now." But this only aggravated Grace still further. Warmly and supportively touching Grace at this moment was not a good idea either. To this, she would often flail at staff and stomp her feet more rebelliously. Reorientation—using logic to orient the person to the current place, time and circumstances—was not an effective intervention for her at these times, because what Grace needed was to be understood. How to do this, though? In her case, the problem was that the staff was interpreting too literally what Grace meant by the word, "home." We normally would understand the word "home" to mean her former place of residence, her house, her hometown. In light of her reactions, though, I suggested to the staff that they might consider other meanings for Grace's pleas. By doing so, the staff was able to relate to Grace and console her. Here's what they did. They said to her, "OK, Grace, let's go home!" One of the nurse's aids would then take Grace back to her room. Why was this effective? It turned out that this is all Grace meant by her "home." As a way of maintaining a sense of permanency and stability, nursing home residents will often consider their room as their new home. Grace was confused about her room location and just needed some directions.

Margaret was another one of my patients who repeated the phrase "I want to go home." She was consoled when she heard others respond, "I would love to hear more about your home, Margaret. Tell me about it, would you?" In hearing this, Margaret would become intensely engaged in describing and reminiscing all about her former life. For her, the word "go" meant "to travel in her mind's eye." A useful way of retraining your ear to better listen and interpret what Alzheimer's sufferers are saying is to practice hearing what they may be saying as if they were speaking in metaphor. From here, all sorts of possible meanings can emerge.

Another way of looking at the words used by Alzheimer's sufferers is to understand that what might be upsetting them may represent an internal rather than an external conflict. Here's what I mean by this. John was a feisty old man with plenty of energy when he needed it, and when the nurses came around with his medication he would fight them before he took it. When a person with Alzheimer's will not cooperate with his caregiver, the conflict may not be so much an interpersonal one between the person and the caregiver but may to a greater degree represent an internal conflict the person may be having inside himself, despite how it might be getting played out with others. For John, the internal conflict had to do with the difficulty he was having in coming to terms with the loss of his independence. You see, John had always lived a very independent life. He was a manager in a steel mill and the patriarch of his family. When he got angry and uncooperative with his nurses it was one way he could externalize the anger he felt at himself for feeling so dependent on others. Other people became targets for the anger he had at himself for needing others and being so dependent. Helping John cope with his anger involved providing him with a vehicle to express just how much he loathed his dependence on others. Once aware of his feelings, he was able to talk about them more directly rather than acting out the internal drama with others. As he did this, his anger at his caregivers diminished, and he became more cooperative in taking his medications.

People with Alzheimer's can have underlying concerns about their own competence: they might have doubts about how well they maintain a helpful role with others, they may feel they lack a sense of purpose, or may feel critical of their ability to care for themselves. Any of these issues can underlie feelings of anger, sadness, fear, and frustration. What's important to recognize about these feelings is that just like the outer bark protects a tree, some feelings are our way of protecting ourselves from more fundamental internal conflicts and dilemmas. Talking with Alzheimer's sufferers means respecting (and not reacting to) their defensiveness. We do this best when we can set aside our own reaction to the other person's feelings. At this point, you might be saying to yourself, "Easier said than done," especially in family relationships with lifelong histories. But with practice, patience, and a recognition that outer actions and words may veil deeper, inner issues, it becomes easier and easier to sit with the feelings of someone with Alzheimer's just long enough to talk about them, work through them, and eventually help the person move past them.

## Talking about Pleasure and Pain

In order to regain our balance from anxiety, distress, or emotional discomfort, understanding hidden feelings and unconscious motives is not always what's important. Sometimes, more than our emotions, it is our thinking and actions that need adjusting.[9] Here's another way to look at it. Many clinicians strongly believe that our thoughts and actions precede or trigger our feelings. Thoughts, actions, and feelings all can be viewed as events that have consequences, either pleasurable or painful. Therefore, healing can occur by increasing pleasurable events and decreasing painful or distressing ones. For example, helping the depressed Alzheimer's sufferer becomes a matter of intentionally increasing the things that bring the person joy and reducing the things that don't.

We might do this with Alzheimer's sufferers by helping them find better ways to relax, to find new hobbies, to increase their opportunity to socialize, or to plan events that reinforce what they enjoy. We might also do this by being mindful of what distresses them and help them to avoid it. Figure 14a presents activities that people with Alzheimer's have stated they find pleasurable.[10] This helps the caregiver to more reliably identify what activities may currently remedy depressive or anxious feelings and what activities from the person's past might be revived to do so. As you read them, I'm sure you'll think of many others.

If you'll recall, I talked earlier about Geraldine, one of my irritable and depressed nursing home patients who had sores so severe they were threatening her life. From the pleasure-pain perspective, Geraldine was depressed because her thoughts about her own worthiness and usefulness were triggers for humiliating feelings of embarrassment, and in order to cope, she isolated herself. Isolation was reinforcing for her because it helped her avoid feeling

**Figure 14a.** How to Identify Pleasant Activities for People with Alzheimer's

For each item, the family member or caregiver can rate each event in two ways:

1. How frequently each event has occurred in the past month (0 = not at all, 1 = a few times, 2 = often), and
2. Whether the event has been or still is enjoyed in the person's life (0 = enjoyed in the past, 1 = enjoys now).

| Pleasant Event | Frequency | Enjoyment |
|---|---|---|
| Being outside (e.g., sitting outside, being in the country) | 0  1  2 | 0  1 |
| Shopping, buying things for themselves and others | 0  1  2 | 0  1 |
| Reading or listening to stories, novels, plays, or poems | 0  1  2 | 0  1 |
| Listing to music | 0  1  2 | 0  1 |
| Watching TV | 0  1  2 | 0  1 |
| Laughing | 0  1  2 | 0  1 |
| Having meals with friends or family (at home or out or on special occasions) | 0  1  2 | 0  1 |
| Making and/or eating snacks | 0  1  2 | 0  1 |
| Helping others, helping around the house (e.g., dusting, cleaning, setting the table, cooking) | 0  1  2 | 0  1 |
| Being with family members (e.g., children, grandchildren, siblings, others) | 0  1  2 | 0  1 |
| Wearing certain clothes (such as new, formal, informal, or favorite clothes) | 0  1  2 | 0  1 |
| Listening to the sounds of nature (e.g., birdsong, wind, surf) | 0  1  2 | 0  1 |
| Getting or sending letters, cards, or notes | 0  1  2 | 0  1 |
| Going on outings (e.g., to the park, on a picnic or barbecue) | 0  1  2 | 0  1 |
| Having coffee, tea, soda, etc. with friends | 0  1  2 | 0  1 |
| Being complimented or told they have done something well | 0  1  2 | 0  1 |
| Exercising (e.g., walking, swimming, aerobics, dancing) | 0  1  2 | 0  1 |
| Going for a ride in the car | 0  1  2 | 0  1 |
| Grooming themselves (e.g., wearing makeup, shaving, having their hair done) | 0  1  2 | 0  1 |
| Recalling and discussing past events | 0  1  2 | 0  1 |

**Figure 14b.** ABC Model for Understanding Behavior

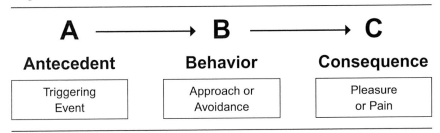

embarrassed and ashamed. The downside was that it made her lonely. In other words, it was just a quick fix. Her trust in me led her to consider that her isolation wasn't really helping her, and on faith she decided to take a risk and tried building her connection with others. Because she found it pleasurable, she began to do it more, and in time she began to see how socializing with others not only made her feel better but helped her avoid feeling lonely and isolated. As a result, her depression lifted. Figure 14b may help you better understand the logic of this approach when talking to people with Alzheimer's. In Geraldine's situation:

A—her thoughts of worthlessness and uselessness were triggers to . . .

B—her isolation, which fostered . . .

C—her loneliness and depressed mood.

My faith in her supported her own faith in herself and fostered her feelings of worthiness. Faith in herself enabled her to risk connecting with others and isolating less. Thinking impairments not withstanding, people with Alzheimer's have a much greater potential that you might think in guiding their own actions, whether they are aware of this potential or not.

## It's All in the Family

People with Alzheimer's are not just individuals but powerful members in a system of family and friends. A family system is composed of a group of relationships, each of which contributes to the family climate, its rhythm, and its pace. When a family member has legal troubles or when one family member decides to marry someone from another race or when a parent dies, the family system as a whole is affected. Just like breaks in the ozone layer affect the climate of our planet, when someone in a family has Alzheimer's it affects the atmosphere in the family system as a whole. Each person in the family system affects the Alzheimer's sufferer, and the Alzheimer's sufferer affects each of them. In essence, family members are part of a network of forces that influence and impact one another.[11]

It has been a remarkable experience for me to witness just how much a person with Alzheimer's picks up on changes in tone and tension in other family members. In a very real sense, Alzheimer's is a family disease, and talking helps a family squarely confront its illness. Bringing key family members together to share what is going well in the care of their afflicted relative, to identify how the family is coping with the situation, to discuss what difficulties are being encountered, to examine what can be done about the problems that are arising, and to explore just how much better a job the family can do to join one another in mutual support are all key elements in improving family communication and care.[12] Here's an example.

Robert was not happy when he was placed in a nursing home. He was in a new and very strange place, and for his protection an ankle monitor was secured to his leg so that he could not elope from the care facility. He did not adjust well to his new surroundings and was angry and uncooperative with the staff. Most nursing home residents eventually settle in and adopt the nursing home as their own, but with Robert this didn't happen. What made it more difficult for Robert was that his family was sharply divided about his placement there, and when they visited him they often argued openly about it in his presence. Robert tried to swallow and assimilate the family's ambivalence and turmoil, and he couldn't do it. My role became to work with his family for a series of family sessions. In the process, a few things became apparent. All the children agreed that the nursing home placement was necessary, but some of them were having a great deal of difficulty resolving their own grief over the loss of their father as they had known him—especially in their loss of him as the head of their household. With mutual understanding and empathy, however, the family as a whole was eventually able to emotionally support its more grief-stricken members and collectively mourn its loss. Not long after this, Robert began to settle in to his new home.

## The Burden on Caregivers

Caregiver burden can affect anyone who is a helping hand to the Alzheimer's patient, but the stress of caregiving is often the greatest in spouses—those who have spent much of their lives with a person who they deeply love but is now behaving in a way that is much different than they ever have. Those who are close to the person with Alzheimer's may not be so willing to acknowledge that caring for their loved one is challenging, stressful, or, at times, even burdensome. They might believe it is "weak" to admit this, or they might believe it is shameful to acknowledge it. Without some recognition of the difficulty, caregivers can unknowingly be affected by the stress of their role, and this can take its toll. Without being addressed, the burden of caregiving can turn into depression, which can affect a caregiver's physical health, which frequently diminishes their feelings of competence in their caregiving role, and which, in turn, can exacerbate further suppression or repression of the felt burden. One of the greatest keys to addressing this spiraling cycle is *rest:*

- ◆ *Physical rest*—getting enough sleep, pacing yourself, not pushing yourself beyond your limits, and keeping your body fit and limber.
- ◆ *Psychological rest*—leisure, meditation, reflection, enjoyable and meaningful conversations with others, and professional counseling if needed.
- ◆ *Spiritual rest*—avoiding self-criticism, being kind to yourself, connecting with others who feed and nurture your soul.

Figure 14c presents a list of feelings and thoughts that family members often experience when their loved one is stricken with Alzheimer's, as well as statements that reflect how caregivers often feel about their role and the stress stemming from that role. These statements have been combined by researchers to create a scale to measure the burden they may be experiencing in their role as caregivers. It's been shown that feelings of caregiver burden are correlated not with the severity of the loved one's illness but with the amount and quality of social support available to the caregiver. What this means is that the amount of burden family caregivers feel does not depend on how ill the stricken member is but instead depends on how much the family feels supported by one another.[13]

In this chapter, I have discussed a variety of methods to deepen communication with the Alzheimer's sufferer. Based on these approaches, I've created a set of guidelines for caregivers when dealing with problems of agitation in Alzheimer's, and these are presented in figure 14d. As you read them, consider what ideas and concepts from the last two chapters form the basis for each of the suggestions. For a more detailed set of suggestions on how to deal with aggressive behavior, take a look at appendix B.

**Figure 14c.** A Scale for Assessing Caregiver Burden and Stress

Listed below are questions reflecting how it might feel to take care of a person with Alzheimer's. In the space provided and using the following rating scale, indicate how often you may experience each of the feelings listed. The average score for caregivers is 31, but regardless of your score, talking with someone about your burden is almost always helpful.

0 Never; 1 Rarely; 2 Sometimes; 3 Frequently; 4 Nearly Always

___ 1. Do you feel that your relative asks for more help than (s)he needs?

___ 2. Do you feel that because of the time you spend with your relative that you don't have enough time for yourself?

___ 3. Do you feel stressed between caring for your relative and trying to meet other responsibilities for your family or work?

___ 4. Do you feel embarrassed over your relative's behavior?

___ 5. Do you feel angry when you are around your relative?

___ 6. Do you feel that your relative currently affects your relationship with other family members or friends in a negative way?

___ 7. Are you afraid of what the future holds for your relative?

___ 8. Do you feel your relative is dependent on you?

___ 9. Do you feel strained when you are around your relative?

___ 10. Do you feel your health has suffered because of your involvement with your relative?

___ 11. Do you feel that you don't have as much privacy as you would like because of your relative?

___ 12. Do you feel that your social life has suffered because you are caring for your relative?

___ 13. Do you feel uncomfortable about having friends over because of your relative?

___ 14. Do you feel that your relative seems to expect you to take care of him/her, as if you were the only one (s)he could depend on?

___ 15. Do you feel that you don't have enough money to care for your relative, in addition to the rest of your expenses?

___ 16. Do you feel that you will be unable to take care of your relative much longer?

___ 17. Do you feel you have lost control of your life since your relative's illness?

___ 18. Do you wish you could just leave the care of your relative to someone else?

___ 19. Do you feel uncertain about what to do about your relative?

___ 20. Do you feel you should be doing more for your relative?

___ 21. Do you feel you could do a better job in caring for your relative?

___ 22. Overall, do you feel burdened in caring for your relative?

___ **Total**

*From Zarit, Orr, and Zarit (1985). Used with permission.*

**Figure 14d.** A Short List of Guidelines for the Alzheimer's Caregiver to Deal with Agitation

---

◆ Look at how the person's regular routine may have been disrupted.

◆ Examine how activities may be lacking as a regular part of his day.

◆ Take a look at how your instructions or your agenda for him may be too complicated; keep things simple for him.

◆ Try to identify what in his surroundings may be triggering his behavior.

◆ Gently redirect him into another activity.

◆ Honor his autonomy by being flexible and by providing him with choices.

◆ Consider that the problems you are observing may be a sign of his grief or loss.

◆ Consider that what you are seeing may be a sign of his unsettling confusion. Reminisce with him about the pleasant events from his past.

◆ Imagine that his agitation may represent his way of acting out a struggle from within himself or from within the family system.

---

## Methods to Build/Maintain Memory

**Spaced Retrieval.** Beatrice was a lovely woman who lived in a nursing home where I provided psychotherapy services. But Beatrice was fretful and anxious, and her memory was failing her. She paced. She ruminated. She'd take her problems to the staff but could not be consoled. I began to see her for weekly psychotherapy, and in our conversations I learned that what worried her the most was being unable to see her children. I commiserated with her loss, and she felt understood. This calmed her to know that she did not have to face her loss alone. It turned out, though, that her children visited her every week—some weeks it was on a weekday, other weeks on the weekend. Beatrice would get overjoyed when she heard that her kids were coming to see her, but she couldn't remember this in between their visits. But despite her children actively being in her life, Beatrice could not remember this and longed for her seemingly lost connection with them.

I assessed the extent of her memory problems in more detail and learned that her memory for new information lasted about ten minutes; then it was gone. I had just been reading, though, about a memory method that increased the time interval for retention in patients with Alzheimer's—so I thought would try it. It's called *spaced retrieval training*.[14] It turns out that if a is reinforced anytime within the retention interval (for Beatrice, minutes), then the retention interval increases. Increase the re enough and the memory eventually gets stored in long-term memory. As we discussed earlier, deficits in long-term memory are generally present in Alzheimer's disease only in the later stages of the illness.

So, what I did was I arranged with Beatrice's kids to place a calendar on her wall that they would sign each day they came to see her. I then began working with Beatrice—I told her about the calendar, and she was excited about it. I then wrote on a card that was permanently placed on her tray table that said, "LONELY FOR THE KIDS? LOOK ON YOUR CALENDAR!" And I trained her with the spaced retrieval method to pick up the card when she was lonely for them. As her memory training proceeded, Beatrice remembered for longer and longer periods of time to pick up the card on her tray table whenever she was lonely. Eventually, the directive to pick up the card became permanently stored in her long-term memory. Once it was, Beatrice could address her own loneliness, and her anxiety and fretfulness resolved.

**Contextual Support.** Another method for facilitating memory is to provide *contextual support* in conversations. Contextual support involves providing additional cues to jog the memory of the Alzheimer's patient. Here's what I mean: asking someone with Alzheimer's, "What's new?" provides less context cues than to ask them, "Did you enjoy Sarah's wedding?" Context cues guide the person to reconnect to their own memory, because they provide the person with a more vivid context within which to recall it.

**Other Techniques.** Other techniques for facilitating recall are to

- slow your rate of speech,
- use common words,
- repeat and rephrase,
- simplify syntax, and
- use YES/NO or forced choice questions.

what they want for dinner is a more difficult s than to ask them if they want chicken or beef. ethod to close a sale. To take another example, mer's, "The meal was prepared by the chef" is ntax than to say, "The chef prepared the meal." ve voice; the second phrase uses an active voice. ulating recall is to create a *sample memory book.*[15] s from the person's past portrayed in words and pictures—who they are, who they are related to, where they lived, what hobbies they enjoyed, milestone events in their life, and so forth—in other words, their identity! This can be a powerful tool to stimulate memory, to calm anxiety, and for many other purposes, and it is shown in figure 14e.

Finally, a note about early detection of memory problems. It is well known that we remember and learn on different levels. On one level, we can remember details of a message we read or are told, and on another level, we can also understand and recall the *gist* of the message—that is, what the message means to us, its global or broader implication. Researchers have discovered that

**Figure 14e.** A Sample Memory Book

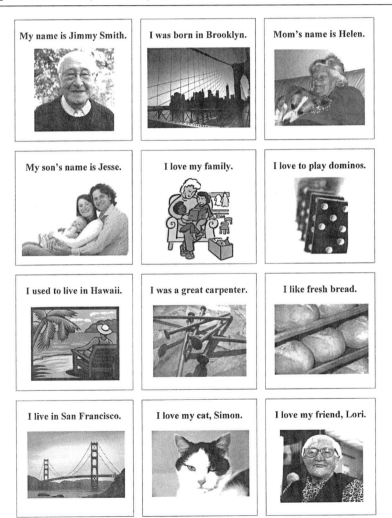

gist-level processing errors may actually precede impairments in memory for specific details and may be an important early marker for cognitive decline.[16]

Talking to people with Alzheimer's has a lot to do with loving them and keeping them safe—loving them not in a romantic way, not in a familial way, not even like a friend—but loving them and keeping them safe as you would anyone who depended on you. The Dalai Lama has said, "My religion is simple. My religion is kindness." This means being kind in the face of frustration, supportive in the face of despair, and by helping Alzheimer's sufferers believe that their most vulnerable and unprotected thoughts and feelings are safe in your mouth.

# 15

## Preventive Activities for Ourselves and Others: Lowering Our Odds of Getting Alzheimer's

"We do not possess our home, our children, or even our body. They are only given to us for a short while to treat with care and respect."

We've come a long way since 1900. Back then, we could expect to live to be about 47 years old. As a society, we've overcome pneumonia, smallpox, and tuberculosis. So much of what determines how long we live nowadays is what we do with our bodies—how we eat, how we exercise, how much rest we get, how we manage our stress. Are there ways we can prevent Alzheimer's disease, though? Yes. Research is showing us that we can lower our odds of getting the disease, delay its onset, and minimize its impact.[1] Because cerebral blood flow decreases with age, much of what we can do to prevent Alzheimer's centers on keeping our blood flowing as freely as possible.[2]

**Keep Physically Active**—Did you know that the brain uses 25 percent of all the oxygen in the body? The medical community has long recognized the impact that physical exercise can have on reducing stress, easing depression, and boosting circulation to vital organs. Its impact on Alzheimer's is also now being appreciated. Any activity that keeps the brain fully oxygenated will optimize its functioning. Overall, exercise is considered to be the single most important contributor to healthful aging. Guidelines recommend at least 30 minutes of moderate-intensity exercise per day.[3]

**Stop Smoking**—Any activity that depletes the brain of oxygen will impair brain functioning and increase the likelihood for Alzheimer's. Smoking, for example, constricts blood vessels, so if you want to guard yourself against developing Alzheimer's, stop smoking.

**Lower Your Cholesterol**—If it makes sense to keep your heart vessels clear, the same can be said for your brain. A growing body of research supports the link between cholesterol and Alzheimer's disease.[4]

**Limit Alcohol Use**—Alcohol, used sensibly and in moderation, is believed to open blood vessels and is part of the MIND diet discussed in chapter 12. Moderation is defined as the consumption of one drink per day for women and up to two drinks per day for men.[5] Regarding alcohol, as with any drug, speak with your physician about it.

**Lower Your Stress**—We know that stress weakens many organs in the body. Research has shown that lowering stress and maintaining a positive outlook can be another important Alzheimer's preventive. A follow-up to the nun study, described in chapter 1, found that the sisters who wrote words like "joy" and "thankful" in their autobiographies lived up to ten years longer than those who expressed more pessimism and other unpleasant attitudes.[6]

**Keep Mentally Active**—My friends Rita and Donna have told me that playing video games of strategy quickens their thinking and prevents Alzheimer's. Whatever changes we can expect as we get older, what we don't use, we lose! Researchers have called this the disuse syndrome. If we don't exercise enough, our muscles get weaker. The same can be said for our thinking. From the person with mild cognitive impairment living at home, to the Alzheimer's patient living in a nursing home, the need to stimulate thinking and keep the mind active is

**Figure 15a.** Ways to Minimize the Risk and Impact of Alzheimer's

- Keep physically active
- Lower your stress
- Stop smoking
- Lower your cholesterol
- Limit alcohol use
- Keep mentally active
- Maintain social stimulation
- Maintain folic acid levels
- Maintain vitamin B$_{12}$ levels
- Increase antioxidant intake
- Increase omega-3 fatty acids
- Decrease saturated fats
- Maintain a positive attitude
- Use cholinesterase inhibitors as prescribed

universally recognized. Just like physical exercise strengthens the body, mental exercise strengthens the mind. This has recently been dubbed neurobics.[7] Rearranging your desk, doing things with the opposite hand, or taking a new route to work are all examples of neurobic exercises which are believed to be beneficial in warding off the impact of the disease. We don't have any control over the fact that we age; we do have some control, however, in how we age. Regularly reading, doing crossword puzzles, or challenging ourselves with any mentally stimulating activity can delay the onset of Alzheimer's or reduce the severity of its symptoms. I shoot pool. What do you do?

**Increase Antioxidant Use**—As we discussed in chapter 12, increasing intake of antioxidants like vitamins E and C fights off the presence of free radicals, which chew up energy within cells and advance the aging process. Figure 15a presents a summary of ways to minimize the risk and impact of Alzheimer's.

## Activities for Those Who Have Alzheimer's

When people are stricken with Alzheimer's, all they may have left to hold on to are the memories from their past—their laughter, the songs they sang and those that were sung to them, the successes they had, or perhaps that they once could dance and share their joy with others. I think that Freddie the Leaf put it the best:

> "Then what has been the reason for all this?" Freddie continued to question. "Why were we here at all if we only have to fall and die?"
>
> Daniel answered in his matter-of-fact way, "It's been about the sun and the moon. It's been about the happy times together. It's been about the shade and the old people and the children. It's been about colors in fall. It's been about the seasons. Isn't that enough?"[8]

Nursing home activity directors have long known that stimulating activities and an active appreciation for our own past can have remarkable effects in staving off the effects of Alzheimer's. With their help, I have compiled some of the best activities I've seem them use. Here is a sampling of helpful activities designed to stimulate positive memories, enliven the senses, heighten physical coordination, increase spontaneity, foster making wise choices, enhance communication with others, and most importantly, to have fun.[9]

### *Reminiscing Exercises*

- Ask the person to name, recall, or sing songs from her era. I will probably be singing "We All Live in a Yellow Submarine" or "When I'm Sixty-Four."
- Ask the person to remember her first job, her first bike, or her first date.
- Stimulate recall of pleasant events by listing important events from a particular year and asking the person to talk about them. For example, in 1965, Los Angeles Dodgers pitcher Sandy Koufax threw a shutout in the World Series and heavyweight boxer Muhammad Ali knocked out Sonny Liston to retain the heavyweight crown.

### *Exercises to Stimulate Sensory and Motor Functioning*

- With eyes closed, play a game by asking the person to identify gathered objects (e.g., a telephone, an apple, a grocery bag).
- Ask the person to sort cards by numbers, by color, by order, or by suit.
- Ask the person to stack cards into piles of five or ten, or stack checkers by height or color.
- Put together a six-piece or twelve-piece puzzle with her.
- Use flash cards to stimulate word identification and language.
- Ask the person to identify objects just by their silhouettes.
- Ask the person to choose a topic and, with her, build on aspects of it that instill choice—for example, by asking her, "What kind of vegetables do you like best? What is your favorite dinner? What do you like best from the bakery?"[10]

### *Exercises with Music* [11]

- In order to maintain thinking abilities, ask the person to finish song titles like "Home, Home on the . . . Range" or "Swing Low, Sweet . . . Chariot." Then ask her to sing the song with you.
- Ask her to finish song lyrics—for example, "I dream of Jeannie . . .

with the light brown hair," "By the light . . . of the silvery moon," and "Silent night, holy night . . . all is calm, all is bright."

◆ To promote discussion or evoke positive memories, play music for her with certain themes like love, hope, or faith.

◆ In order to maintain physical conditioning, try tossing balloons with her to recorded music or encourage movement to music with scarves or streamers (fast, slow, high, low), or play or sing a familiar song while completing an activity of daily living. Hearing Jiminy Cricket singing "Whistle While You Work" always got me in a good mood.

## Challenge Yourself and Others with Brainteasers

I have an Alzheimer's patient in the early stage of the illness who loves riddles and brainteasers. I recently challenged her with one: "Two men were playing chess. They played five games. Each won three games. There were no ties. How can this be?" She sat and thought about the puzzle, then a smile came over her face. She then said, "Because they weren't playing each other!" In Eastern thought, it is considered meditative to imagine the sound of one hand clapping. It is meditative because it challenges the mind to search itself for an answer it cannot find. Peace comes when you can search for something and at the same time be patient with yourself that you have not found it. What matters in meditation is the search. It's calming because our mind is focused. The same is true for activities that entertain and challenge the mind of the Alzheimer's sufferer. Here are some examples to try with someone you know.

◆ Name three sports that take place on wheels.
◆ Name a man's name that begins with the letter "O."
◆ Which state has only one syllable?
◆ Which country is below France?

Success at activities like these can build confidence and enhance pride while stimulating neural connections that can help the Alzheimer's sufferer maintain thinking abilities.

## Activities to Stimulate Socialization

The following activities can be useful in a group but can also be adapted for one-on-one use at home.

- Ask the person to disclose information about herself—for example, you could ask her to respond to the following sentence completion stems:
  - One thing I do well is . . .
  - One thing that amuses me is . . .
  - One thing I would like to be remembered for is . . .
- To encourage movement and livelier interactive exchanges, ask people to find someone in the group who, for example, likes ice cream, plays a musical instrument, or has traveled out of the country.
- Invite the person to read a book with you or read it to her.
- Read the day's newspaper and ask her to discuss it with you.
- Invite her to play bingo or trivia games or create a crafts project.
- Challenge her to a spelling bee, to tell a story about herself, or to complete a simple crossword puzzle.

Taking care of ourselves is essential for optimal living. We have only one chance with our mind and body. If we do this for ourselves and if we help others do it for themselves, we are doing what we can to fend off the impact of this mind-stealing, deadly disease.

# Appendix A

## Additional Resources and Information on Alzheimer's Dementia

Administration on Aging
Washington, DC 20201
(800) 677-1116
www.aoa.gov

Alzheimer's Association
National Headquarters
225 N. Michigan Ave., Floor 17
Chicago, IL 60611-7633
(800) 272-3900
www.alz.org

The Alzheimer's Store
12633 159th Court North
Jupiter, FL 33478
www.alzstore.com

Alzheimer Society of Canada
20 Eglinton Ave. West, 16th Floor
Toronto, Ontario M4R 1K8
Canada
(800) 616-8816
www.alzheimer.ca/en

Family Caregiver Alliance
785 Market St., Suite 750
San Francisco, CA 94103
(800) 445-8106
www.caregiver.org

Gerontology Society of America
1220 L Street NW, Suite 901
Washington, DC 20005
(202) 842-1275
www.geron.org

National Council on Aging
251 18th St. South, Suite 500
Arlington, VA 22202
(571) 527-3900
www.ncoa.org

National Hospice and Palliative
Care Organization
1731 King St.
Alexandria, VA 22314
(703) 837-1500
www.nhpco.org

National Institute of Mental Health
Science Writing, Press, and
Dissemination Branch
6001 Executive Blvd.
Room 8184, MSC 9663
Bethesda, MD 20892-9663
(866) 615-6464
www.nimh.nih.gov

National Institute on Aging
Building 31, Room 5C27
31 Center Drive, MSC 2292
Bethesda, MD 20892
(800) 222-2225
www.nia.nih.gov/

# Appendix B

## What to Do about Aggressive Behavior

Hearing rude or abrasive remarks from the very person you are trying to help is one of the most difficult aspects of caregiving. Understanding and knowing how to better handle what may be going on in these situations can bring a sense of order and calm to an upsetting experience and can reduce stress and improve the living climate for all concerned.

All of us have our limits, especially when it comes to tolerating aggressive behavior. As a caregiver, after your best efforts have been exhausted, you may feel angry or hurt or afraid. You may find yourself trying to impose the "rule of law" or you may find yourself unintentionally using cutting or angry words to regain control of a situation. You may even try to shame the person into submission. Although you might get what you want in the short run, these methods will generally be ineffective, because in the long run they are more likely to damage the relationship by evoking guilt, remorse, and resentments on both sides. So when you need cooperation in future situations you'll be less likely to get it.

What's most important in altering aggressive behavior in people with Alzheimer's is to keep your cool long enough to figure out what the real problem is. Here are some tips:[1]

Before you do anything, make sure you keep a safe distance from the person. To help keep someone else safe, you need to first keep yourself safe. Once you do this, you can better judge what might be done next. Your next step is to cool down the situation. Using a calm and reassuring tone of voice, the goal here is to "turn down the volume" on the situation. You will not get what you want if you or the other person is upset. The calmer you can make the situation, the more likely you will be able to identify the triggers or causes of the abrasive or aggressive behavior—and this is ultimately the key. Here are some ideas on how to begin this process:

Try to rebuild trust—this can be done by calmly reassuring the person that you want to know what may be upsetting him. People will often feed off your feelings. If you are calm, they will more likely be calm; if your feelings are escalating, theirs will, too. Being calm is what fosters control in the situation. Let them feed off your serenity.

Really listen to him—try to understand the meaning behind what the person is saying. Find out what may have triggered his aggressive reaction. Try to understand him before you ask him to understand you. By doing this, he will be more receptive and willing to hear what you have to say.

At some point you will need to tell the person calmly but firmly how his reaction to the situation isn't helping him, why it isn't helping him, and some reasonable limits that need to be set. Let him know how his aggressive reaction keeps you from helping him solve his problem. For example, you can point out how his aggressive behavior has increased lately, the impact it is having on others, how it might be distressful for the person himself, and why it needs to stop. You might say in a gentle and caring way,

- "Mom, you have been yelling more lately. I can see things are upsetting to you . . . but you need to stop yelling."
- "Dad, I know you are upset, but as we've told you before, yelling is not the answer (or . . . is not allowed here)."
- "When you yell at others, Vivian, it can anger or startle them. This is not what others want."
- When the person is clear on the consequences of his actions, you might say, "As we have said before, Grampa, if you continue this behavior it will be more difficult for me to talk with you."
- For very severe and repetitive aggressive behavior, you might say, "Aurianna, as we have discussed with you before, if you continue to hit me you will begin to lose some of your special privileges."

You will now be in a better position to rechannel the person's actions in a more constructive direction. A good way to do this is to instruct the person in advance exactly what you want him to do and avoid telling him what you don't want him to do. Do not attempt to physically force him to do what you want. If the person continues to exhibit physically aggressive behavior and will not take your redirection, it is time to get help from others. Abrasive or aggressive behaviors are very difficult problems to curb, and it often takes more than one person for some people to get the message. You might say, "I am coming in to clean your room now, Michael. Remember, I want you to react calmly," or "Miles, I will need to come near your bed now. I want you to keep your hands to yourself. Will you do that for me?"

If things don't work out the way you had hoped or your interventions are only partially effective, let the situation cool down before you try again. If the aggressive behavior persists, keep your cool. Don't let yourself get too frustrated. Walk away, leave the area, and let some time pass before you return. Review your plan. When you do return you will be more emotionally centered to calmly reiterate and reinforce your message. Once you sense any success at all, though, show the person you appreciate what she has done. When the person begins to do the right thing she needs to know it and feel good about what she has done. You can do this with words or actions—anything that might communicate to her that you care about her and appreciate what she has just done. This will help you get more cooperation from her in the future.

Keep track of how often and when the problem occurs. Doing this will help you discover any patterns in the person's actions that reveal what might be triggering her aggressive behavior. Does the behavior happen mostly at night? When others are around? When the person is anxious or hurt? Might it have been unintentionally triggered by something you did or said? This can give you some power in predicting when the behavior might occur again. Once you discover any patterns in her behavior, try in advance to prompt her to behave in the way you need. For example, if mealtime is a chronic problem time for the person, let her know in advance that the problem might arise and what you want her to do instead.

Sometimes a simple distraction technique can work best. For example, you might find it helpful to say in a loving and caring way, "Mr. Robinson, you are yelling again . . . you agreed not to do that . . . why don't you tell me a little more about those nights you spent shooting pool." Another method you can use is to provide some freedom and space for the person to discharge or vent her underlying feelings in advance of her acting them out aggressively. Sometimes, aggressive behavior is triggered by anger, but it also can be triggered by anxiety, loneliness, frustration, or any other feeling. If you feel the person may be yelling at others because she is lonely, when things have cooled down ask her to talk to you about those feelings.

Clarifying and organizing your ideas into a plan can be helpful for you, the other person, other caregivers—everyone. If you find yourself losing your cool too often, though, ask others how they handle the situation. If you find that your care recipient's aggressive behavior pushes your buttons, join the club—it happens to all of us. Don't stop there, though. Talk to others about how they deal with the problem. There is no shame in getting your buttons pushed—what you want to avoid is bottling up those feelings.

# Appendix C

## Effective Uses of Psychological Interventions in Long-Term Care Facilities[1]

The question of placing someone with Alzheimer's in a nursing home is a difficult one. Nearly half of those who suffer from the disorder, however, live in the community—frequently with spouses, other family members, or tragically alone. Although the benefits of community living cannot be ignored, making the decision to place a loved one in a nursing home must weigh the importance of honoring the person's need for autonomy and independence with a realistic assessment of his safety, medical needs, and the stress incurred by his home caregivers.

Research has shown that about 70 percent of assisted living residents and nursing home residents have some type of dementia. About 50 percent of people newly relocated to long-term care facilities are at a heightened risk for depression, and over 40 percent of all residents in long-term care can be diagnosed with some type of mood or anxiety disorder. Mental health problems such as these can worsen the status of a person's overall health condition which, in turn, can divert attention away from underlying psychological causes. For example, stress increases the risk for coronary heart disease and suppresses the immune response, depression can lead to increased mortality from heart disease and cancer, and mood disorders can contribute to excessive disability in people with Alzheimer's.

Because elderly nursing home residents are more likely to report bodily symptoms than emotional ones, mood disorders in these residents are often underdiagnosed. Most long-term care programs are designed primarily to aid older adults with chronic physical disabilities or impairments in thinking but often fail to adequately address impairments in mood and behavior. The consequences of underdiagnosed mental health issues, however, can be severe. Elderly people with sleep and appetite disturbances symptomatic of depression have been shown to be at an increased risk for dementia, impairments in functional abilities, and premature death.

In 1987, the Federal Nursing Home Reform Act of the Omnibus Budget Reconciliation Act asserted that all interventions in the nursing home must be guided by using the lowest level of chemical or physical restraint possible. This meant that psychological and social interventions were recommended before the use of physical and chemical restraints. Unfortunately, when treating mood or behavior problems, the surgeon general has found that too frequently the first course of treatment in long-term care facilities is medication. Research has shown that for many mental disorders, medicines are no more effective than counseling. Furthermore, for those mental disorders for which medications may be appropriate, the simultaneous use of counseling and medicines is generally more effective than the use of medicines alone.

Counseling and social interventions may be the treatment of choice for many older nursing home residents, particularly for those who are unable to tolerate or prefer not to take medication or who are confronting stressful situations with insufficient social support. Counseling and social interventions in long-term care facilities not only can help relieve the symptoms of many mental disorders but can also strengthen a person's ability to cope, encourage compliance with medications, and generally promote healthy behavior. At minimum, assisted living and nursing home residents should be screened for depression and dementia.

# Appendix D

## Additional Tables and Figures

**Table 1.** Emotional Signs and Symptoms That Accompany Alzheimer's

| Type of Problem | Frequency in Alzheimer's Sufferers |
| --- | :---: |
| Apathy and lethargy | 72% |
| Delusions | 70% |
| Aggression and agitation | 60% |
| Anxiety and excessive worry | 48% |
| Psychomotor disturbances | 46% |
| Irritability | 42% |
| Sleep disturbances | 42% |
| Depression | 38% |
| Disinhibition | 36% |
| Sundowning | 18% |
| Hallucinations | 15% |
| Hypersexuality | 3% |
| Euphoria | 2% |
| Obsessions or compulsions | 2% |

From Scharre (1999). Used with permission.

**Table 2.** Distinctions between Alzheimer's and Delirium

| Characteristic | Delirium | Alzheimer's |
| --- | --- | --- |
| Onset (the single most important distinction) | Short | Gradual |
| Attention deficits (the second most important distinction) | Always present | Usually absent |
| Impaired memory, thinking, and judgment | Always present | Always present |
| Fluctuation of symptoms over the course of the day | Always present | Occasionally present |
| Disorientation (usually to time or place) | Always present | Usually present |
| Vivid perceptual disturbances | Usually present | Occasionally present |
| Incoherent speech | Usually present | Occasionally present |
| Disrupted sleep-wake cycle | Usually present | Occasionally present |
| Gets worse at night | Usually present | Occasionally present |

Adapted from Liston (1984). Used with permission.

**Table 3.** Distinctions between Cortical and Subcortical Dementia

| Characteristic | Subcortical Dementia (like Parkinson's) | Cortical Dementia (like Alzheimer's) |
|---|---|---|
| Speech | Abnormal | Normal until late in the disease |
| Memory | Forgetful | Impaired learning |
| Calculation ability | Preserved until late in the disease | Involved early |
| Mood | Depressed, particularly early in the disease | Often depressed but more prevalent in the early stages of the disease |
| Coordination | Impaired | Normal until late in the disease |
| Motor speed and control | Slowed | Normal |

Adapted from J. L. Cummings and D. F. Benson, *Dementia: A Clinical Approach,* 2nd ed. Copyright © 1992. Reprinted with permission from Butterworth-Heinemann; and A. K. Pajeau and G. C. Roman, "HIV Encephalopathy and Dementia," in *The Psychiatric Clinics of North America: The Interface of Psychiatry and Neurology,* vol. 15, 455–66. Copyright © 1992. Reprinted with permission from W. B. Saunders Company.

**Table 4.** Features Useful in Differentiating Alzheimer's Disease from Dementia Syndrome of Depression

| Measure | Alzheimer's Disease | Dementia Syndrome of Depression |
|---|---|---|
| Duration | Long | Short |
| Psychiatric history | Unusual | Usual |
| Progression | Slow | Rapid |
| Complaints of deficits | Variable and nonspecific | Abundant and specific |
| Emotional reaction | Variable | Marked distress |
| Person's evaluation of accomplishments | Variable | Minimized or diminished |
| Behavioral consistency with cognitive deficits | Usual | Unusual |
| Delusions | Independent of mood | Consistent with mood |
| Mood disorder | Environmentally responsive | Persistent |
| Recognition memory | Impaired | Relatively intact |
| Making up answers when they don't know | More often | Less often |
| Performance effort | Good | Poor |
| Performance on tasks of similar difficulty | Consistent | Variable |
| Prompting | Less helpful | Helpful |
| Awareness of impairment | Relatively unaware | Relatively aware |

Adapted from J. L. Cummings and D. F. Benson, *Dementia: A Clinical Approach,* 2nd ed. Copyright © 1992. Reprinted with permission from Butterworth-Heinemann; and A. K. Pajeau and G. C. Roman, "HIV Encephalopathy and Dementia," in *The Psychiatric Clinics of North America: The Interface of Psychiatry and Neurology* 15 (1992): 455–66. Copyright © 1992. Reprinted with permission from W. B. Saunders Company.

**Table 5.** Medications That Commonly Cause Confusion

| Class | Use | Examples of More Problematic Medications |
|---|---|---|
| Anticholinergics | Block the action of the neurotransmitter acetylcholine | Atropine, scopolamine, and many antihistamines, such as chlorpheniramine, cyproheptadine, dexchlorpheniramine, diphenhydramine, hydroxyzine, promethazine |
| Antidepressants | Depression | Amitriptyline, doxepin |
| Antiparkinson drugs | Parkinson's disease symptoms | Levodopa (L-dopa or sinemet), bromocriptine |
| Antipsychotics | Hallucinations, delusions | Chlorpromazine, haloperidol, thioridazine, thiothixene |
| Barbiturates | Sleep and anxiety | Phenobarbital, secobarbital |
| Benzodiazepines | Sleep and anxiety | Chlordiazepoxide, diazepam, flurazepam, nitrazepam |
| Histamine-2 (H2) blockers | Block the action of gastric acid secretion | Cimetidine, famotidine, nizatidine, ranitidine |
| Non-steroidal anti-inflammatory drugs (NSAIDs) | Pain | Ibuprofen, indomethacin |
| Opioids | Pain | Morphine, propoxyphene, meperidine |
| Steroids | Inflammation, pulmonary disease | Prednisone, dexamethasone, methylprednisolone |

**Figure 1.** How Clinicians Can Differentiate between Alzheimer's Disease and Vascular Dementia

| Features | Score |
|---|---|
| Abrupt onset | 2 |
| Stepwise deterioration | 1 |
| Fluctuating course | 2 |
| Nocturnal confusion | 1 |
| Relative preservation of personality | 1 |
| Depression | 1 |
| Somatic complaints | 1 |
| Emotional incontinence | 1 |
| History of hypertension | 1 |
| History of strokes | 2 |
| Evidence of associated atherosclerosis | 1 |
| Focal neurological signs | 2 |
| Focal neurological symptoms | 2 |

*Scores of 1–4:* Suggest Alzheimer's disease
*Scores of 7–18:* Suggest vascular dementia
*Scores 4 and 7:* Indeterminate/mixed cases

*Reprinted with the permission of The Free Press, a Division of Simon & Schuster Adult Publishing Group, from V. C. Hachinski, "Differential Diagnosis of Alzheimer's Dementia: Multi-infarct Dementia," in B. Reisberg, ed.,* Alzheimer's Disease: The Standard Reference *(pp. 188–92). Copyright © 1983. All rights reserved.*

**Figure 2.** The Standard Comprehensive Workup for Delirium and Alzheimer's Dementia

| Workup | Delirium | Alzheimer's Dementia |
|---|:---:|:---:|
| **Exams** | | |
| Neurological exam | ✓ | ✓ |
| Vitals | ✓ | ✓ |
| Mental status | ✓ | ✓ |
| Review of medications | ✓ | ✓ |
| **Laboratory Tests** | | |
| Complete blood count | ✓ | ✓ |
| Blood chemistry | ✓ | ✓ |
| Thyroid function | ✓ | ✓ |
| HIV test | ✓ | ✓ |
| Urinalysis | ✓ | ✓ |
| Electrocardiogram | ✓ | ✓ |
| Electroencephalograph | ✓ | ✓ |
| Chest X-ray | ✓ | ✓ |
| Alcohol and drug screen | ✓ | ✓ |
| **Imaging Methods** | | |
| Positron emission tomography (PET) | ✓ | ✓ |
| Single photon emission computed tomography (SPECT) | ✓ | ✓ |
| Functional magnetic resonance imagery (fMRI) | ✓ | ✓ |
| **Other Tests** | | |
| $B_{12}$ | ✓ | ✓ |
| Folic acid | ✓ | ✓ |
| Corticosteroids | ✓ | |
| Arterial blood gases | | ✓ |
| Genotyping | | ✓ |
| apolipoprotein-E[†] | | |
| tau[†] | | |
| amyloid precursor protein[†] | | |
| presenilin-1[‡] | | |
| presenilin-2[†] | | |

[†]Available for diagnostic confirmation only.
[‡]Available for diagnostic and predictive purposes.

**Figure 3.** Categories of the Full Mental Status Exam

◆ Alertness

◆ Orientation

◆ Appearance and Behavior

◆ Reliability, Honesty, and Accuracy

◆ Speech

   *Rate, Rhythm, Volume*

   *Pace, Manner, Phraseology*

◆ Attention Span

◆ Concentration

◆ Agnosia

◆ Apraxia

◆ Aphasia

◆ Executive Functioning

   *Abstract Reasoning*

   *Planning, Organizing, Sequencing*

◆ Memory

   *Immediate*

   *Short-Term*

   *Long-Term*

◆ Fund of Information and Intelligence

◆ Psychotic Processes

   *Hallucinations*

   *Delusions*

   *Stream of Thought*

◆ Thought Content

   *Obsessions*

   *Compulsions*

   *Fears, Phobias*

   *Irritability, Anger*

   *Sadness, Loneliness*

   *Guilt, Shame*

   *Somatic Concerns*

◆ Substance Abuse

◆ Mood

   *Depression*

   *Suicidal/Homicidal Inclinations*

   *Anxiety and Panic*

   *Mania*

◆ Affect (the level and range of emotion)

◆ Judgment and Insight

◆ Self-Image

◆ Coping Style and Abilities

◆ Personality Features

**Figure 4.** The Hopkins Competency Assessment Test

| Questions | Appropriate Answers |
|---|---|
| What are the four things a doctor must tell a person before beginning a procedure? | *a. What the doctor is going to do.*<br>*b. What could go right.*<br>*c. What could to wrong.*<br>*d. What else the doctor could do instead.* |
| True or false: After learning about the procedure, the person can decide not to have the procedure done. | *True.* |
| What can sometimes happen to the thinking of a person who has been sick for a long time? | *After a while, the person's thinking may not be as good as it is now.* |
| Finish the sentence: A person whose thinking gets bad may not be able to _____. | *Tell the doctor what the person wants done.* |
| What two things should people tell their doctor and family before their thinking gets bad? | *The person should write down who else the doctor can talk to in order to make medical decisions for them.* |
| What are these instructions to doctors and family called? | *They are called durable powers of attorney.* |
| Score 1 point for each correct answer. Ten points are possible.<br>Scores of 3 out of 10 or less indicate incompetency with 100% accuracy. | |

*Reprinted with permission from J. S. Janofsky, R. J. McCarthy, and M. F. Folstein, "The Hopkins Competency Assessment Test: A Brief Method for Evaluating Patients' Capacity to Give Informed Consent,"* Hospital and Community Psychiatry, *43 (1992): 132–35. Copyright © 1992, American Psychiatric Association.*

**Figure 5.** The Cornell Scale for Depression in Dementia

This measurement instrument is used by professionals who have observed the person with Alzheimer's in the week just prior to the rating. No score should be given if symptoms result from a physical disability or illness other than dementia.

### Scoring System
A = Unable to evaluate
0 = Absent
1 = Mild to intermittent
2 = Severe

| | A | 0 | 1 | 2 |
|---|---|---|---|---|
| **A. Mood-Related Signs** | | | | |
| 1. Anxiety, anxious expressions, rumination, worrying | | | | |
| 2. Sadness, sad expressions, sad voice, tearfulness | | | | |
| 3. Lack of reaction to pleasant events | | | | |
| 4. Irritability, annoyed, short temper | | | | |
| **B. Behavioral Disturbances** | | | | |
| 5. Agitation, restlessness, hand-wringing, hair-pulling | | | | |
| 6. Slow movements, slow speech, slow reactions | | | | |
| 7. Multiple physical complaints (score 0 if gastrointestinal symptoms only) | | | | |
| 8. Loss of interests, less involved in usual activities (score only if change occurred only within the last month) | | | | |
| **C. Physical Signs** | | | | |
| 9. Appetite loss, eating less than usual | | | | |
| 10. Weight loss (score 2 if greater than five pounds in one month) | | | | |
| 11. Lack of energy, fatigued easily, inability to sustain activities | | | | |

**Figure 5.** *(continued)*

This measurement instrument is used by professionals who have observed the person with Alzheimer's in the week just prior to the rating. No score should be given if symptoms result from a physical disability or illness other than dementia.

**Scoring System**

A = Unable to evaluate

0 = Absent

1 = Mild to intermittent

2 = Severe

| | A | 0 | 1 | 2 |
|---|---|---|---|---|
| **D.** *Cyclic Functions* | | | | |
| 1. Daily variation of mood, symptoms worse in the morning | | | | |
| 2. Difficulty falling asleep, falls asleep later than usual | | | | |
| 3. Multiple awakenings during sleep | | | | |
| 4. Early morning awakenings earlier than usual for this individual | | | | |
| **E.** *Ideational Disturbances* | | | | |
| 5. Suicidal, feels life is not worth living | | | | |
| 6. Poor self-esteem, self- blame, self-depreciation, feelings of failure | | | | |
| 7. Pessimism, anticipates the worst | | | | |
| 8. Mood-congruent delusions of poverty, illness, or loss | | | | |

**Total Score:** A score of greater than 12 indicates probable depression.

*Reprinted from George S. Alexopoulos, Robert C. Abrams, Robert C. Young, and Charles A. Shamoian, "Cornell Scale for Depression in Dementia,"* Biological Psychiatry *23 (1988): 271–84. Copyright © 1988, with permission from the Society of Biological Psychiatry.*

# Notes

## Notes to the Preface

1. *Fearless.* Director: Peter Weir. Performers: Jeff Bridges, Isabella Rossellini, Rosie Perez, John Turtourro, Tom Hulce, Benecio Benicio Del Toro. Warner Brothers, 1993.

2. American Psychiatric Association, *Diagnostic and Statistical Manual of Mental Disorders,* 5th ed. (Washington, DC: American Psychiatric Association, 2013); H. I. Kaplan and B. J. Saddock, eds., *Synopsis of Psychiatry* (Baltimore: Williams and Wilkins, 1994).

## Notes to the Second Edition Introduction

1. B. D. Carpenter et al., "Reaction to a Dementia Diagnosis in Individuals with Alzheimer's Disease and Mild Cognitive Impairment," *Journal of the American Geriatrics Society* 56 (2008): 405–12.

2. A. S. Kelly et al., "The Burden of Health Care Costs for Patients with Dementia in the Last 5 Years of Life," *Annals of Internal Medicine* 163 (2015): 729–36.

## Notes to Chapter 1

1. Unless otherwise referenced, each chapter begins with a quote from Jack Kornfield's *Buddha's Little Instruction Book.* (New York: Bantam, 1994).

2. T. Needels and T. Bilanow, "Power Up Your Brain," *Psychology Today,* August 2002, 44–51.

3. C. M. Cowles, ed., *2001 Nursing Home Statistical Yearbook* (Montgomery Village, MD: Cowles Research Group, 2002).

4. T. DeBaggio, *Losing My Mind: An Intimate Look at Life with Alzheimer's* (New York: Simon & Shuster Audio, 2002).

5. K. Steenland et al., "A Meta-Analysis of Alzheimer's Disease Incidence and Prevalence

Comparing African-Americans and Caucasians," *Journal of Alzheimer's Disease* 50, no. 1 (2015): 1–6.

6. Alzheimer's Association, "2015 Alzheimer's Disease Facts and Figures," *Alzheimer's & Dementia: The Journal of the Alzheimer's Association* 11, no. 3 (2015): 332. See also J. C. Chen, S. Borson, and J. M. Scanlan, "Stage-Specific Prevalence of Behavioral Symptoms in Alzheimer's Disease in a Multi-ethnic Sample," *American Journal of Geriatric Psychiatry* 8 (2000): 123–33.

7. J. L. Tsai and L. L. Carstensen, "Clinical Intervention with Ethnic Minority Elders," in *The Practical Handbook of Clinical Gerontology,* ed. L. L. Carstensen, B. A. Edelstein, and L. Dornbrand (Thousand Oaks, CA: Sage, 1996), 76–106.

8. C. G. Lyketsos, "Current Issues in Dementia Care," *Audio Digest Psychiatry* 33, no. 18 (21 September 2004).

9. C. M. Callahan, H. C. Hendrie, and W. M. Tierney, "Documentation and Evaluation of Cognitive Impairment in Elderly Primary Care Patients," *Annals of Internal Medicine* 122 (1995): 422–29.

10. U.S. Department of Health and Human Services, *Mental Health: A Report of the Surgeon General* (Rockville, MD: U.S. Department of Health and Human Services, 1999). Available online at https://profiles.nlm.nih.gov/ps/access/NNBBHS.pdf.

11. J. C. Breitner, "Clinical Genetics and Genetic Counseling in Alzheimer's Disease," *Annals of Internal Medicine* 115 (1991): 601–6.

12. J. Cummings and D. Jeste, "Alzheimer's Disease and Its Management in the Year 2010," *Psychiatric Services* 50 (1999): 1173–77.

13. C. G. Lyketsos, "Current Issues in Dementia Care."

14. D. Snowdon, *Aging with Grace: What the Nun Study Teaches Us about Leading Longer, Healthier and More Meaningful Lives* (New York: Bantam, 2001).

15. C. E. Coffey et al., "Relation of Education to Brain Size in Normal Aging: Implications for the Reserve Hypothesis," *Neurology* 53 (1999): 189–96.

16. B. Schmand et al., "The Effects of Intelligence and Education on the Development of Dementia: A Test of the Brain Reserve Hypothesis," *Psychological Medicine* 27 (1997): 1337–44.

## Notes to Chapter 2

1. American Psychological Association, "Reports of the Association: Guidelines for the Evaluation of Dementia and Age-Related Cognitive Decline," *American Psychologist* 53 (1998): 1298–1303.

2. S. K. Whitbourne, "Psychological Perspective on the Normal Aging Process," in *The Practical Handbook of Clinical Gerontology,* ed. L. L. Carstensen, B. A. Edelstein, and L. Dornbrand (Thousand Oaks, CA: Sage, 1996), 3–35.

## Notes to Chapter 3

1. J. R. Youngjohn and T. H. Crook, "Dementia," in *The Practical Handbook of Clinical Gerontology,* ed. L. L. Carstensen, B. A. Edelstein, and L. Dornbrand (Thousand Oaks, CA: Sage, 1996), 76–106.

2. C. G. Lyketsos, "Current Issues in Dementia Care," *Audio Digest Psychiatry* 33, no. 18 (21 September 2004).

3. R. C. Strub and F. W. Black, *Neurobehavioral Disorders: A Clinical Approach* (Philadelphia: F. A. Davis, 1988).

4. In this context, I am using the DSM-IV criteria for dementia—American Psychiatric Association, *Diagnostic and Statistical Manual of Mental Disorders,* 4th ed. (Washington, DC: American Psychiatric Association, 1994)—because I find it easier to understand. For additional diagnostic methods, see American Psychiatric Association, *Diagnostic and Statistical Manual of Mental Disorders,* 5th ed. (Washington, DC: American Psychiatric Association, 2013) and J. M. Foley and A. L. Heck, "Neurocognitive Disorders in Aging: A Primer on DSM-5 Changes and Framework for Application to Practice," *Clinical Gerontologist* 37, no. 4 (2014), 317–46.

5. Adapted from D. Snowdon, *Aging with Grace: What the Nun Study Teaches Us about Leading Longer, Healthier and More Meaningful Lives* (New York: Bantam, 2001).

6. T. Needels and T. Bilanow, "Power Up Your Brain," *Psychology Today,* August 2002, 44–51.

7. American Psychiatric Association, *Diagnostic and Statistical Manual;* R. E. Markin, *The Alzheimer's Cope Book: The Complete Care Manual for Patients and Their Families* (New York: Citadel Press, 1992); L. N. Mace and P. V. Rabins, *The 36-Hour Day* (Baltimore: Johns Hopkins University Press, 1996).

8. D. Scharre, "Treatment of Dementia," April 26–29, 1999, broadcast of Ohio Medical Education Network.

9. S. H. Zarit, N. K. Orr, and J. M. Zarit, *The Hidden Victims of Alzheimer's Disease: Families Under Stress* (New York: New York University Press, 1985); R. Petersen, ed., *Mayo Clinic on Alzheimer's Disease* (Rochester, MN: Mayo Clinic Health Information, 2002).

10. Lori Tuttle-Kraus (personal communication, June 2003).

## Notes to Chapter 4

1. This is a wonderful old Buddhist expression that I found in E. Bayda, *Being Zen* (Boston: Shambhala, 2002).

2. H. Gruetzner, *Alzheimer's: A Caregiver's Guide and Sourcebook* (New York: Wiley, 1988).

3. This figure was developed from a variety of sources but by no means illustrates the many disorders that can cause dementia-like symptoms. For a more complete list of other medical conditions that can mimic the symptoms of Alzheimer's, see, for example: H. I. Kaplan and B. J. Saddock, eds., *Synopsis of Psychiatry* (Baltimore: Williams and Wilkins, 1994); and E. D. Caine and H. T. Grossman, "Neuropsychiatric Assessment," in *Handbook of Mental Health and Aging,* ed. J. E. Birren, R. B. Sloan, and G. D. Cohen (San Diego: Academic Press, 1992), 603–42.

4. J. R. Youngjohn and T. H. Crook, "Dementia," in *The Practical Handbook of Clinical Gerontology*, eds. L. L. Carstensen, B. A. Edelstein, and L. Dornbrand (Thousand Oaks, CA: Sage, 1996), 76–106; C. J. Golden and A. Chronopolous, "Dementia," in *Handbook of Clinical Geropsychology,* ed. M. Hersen and V. B. Van Hasselt (New York: Plenum, 1998), 113–45.

5. Ibid.

6. To learn more about genetics, visit Genetics Home Reference: Your Guide to Understanding Genetic Conditions at https://ghr.nlm.nih.gov/.

7. A. R. Koudinov and N. V. Koudinova, "Amyloid Beta Protein Restores Hippocampal Long Term Potentiation: A Central Role for Cholesterol?" *Neurobiology of Lipids* 1, no. 8 (2003).

8. J. Chu et al., "Gamma Secretase-Activating Protein Is a Substrate for Caspase-3: Implications for Alzheimer's Disease," *Biological Psychiatry* 77, no. 8 (2015): 720–28. See also A. Gupta and C. Iadecola, "Impaired Aβ Clearance: A Potential Link Between Atherosclerosis and Alzheimer's Disease," *Name: Frontiers in Aging Neuroscience* 7 (2015): 115. See also Y.-H. Suh and F. Checler, "Amyloid Precursor Protein, Presenilins, and Alpha-Synuclein: Molecular Pathogenesis and Pharmacological Applications in Alzheimer's Disease," *Pharmacological Reviews* 54 (2002): 469–525.

9. U.S. Department of Health and Human Services, *Mental Health: A Report of the Surgeon General* (Rockville, MD: U.S. Department of Health and Human Services, 1999). Available online at https://profiles.nlm.nih.gov/ps/access/NNBBHS.pdf. For more information on Alzheimer's disease and genotyping, see R. Duara et al., "Alzheimer's Disease: Interaction of Apolipoprotein E Genotype, Family History of Dementia, Gender, Education, Ethnicity, and Age of Onset," *Neurology* 46 (1996): 1575–79.

10. S. Roeber et al., "Three Novel Presenilin 1 Mutations Marking the Wide Spectrum of Age at Onset and Clinical Patterns in Familial Alzheimer's Disease," *Journal of Neural Transmission* 122, no. 12 (2015): 1715–19.

11. U.S. Department of Health and Human Services, *Mental Health*. See also R. Duara et al., "Alzheimer's Disease."

12. C. Pan et al., "Diagnostic Values of Cerebrospinal Fluid T-Tau and Aβ42 Using Meso Scale Discovery Assays for Alzheimer's Disease," *Journal of Alzheimer's Disease: JAD* 45, no. 3 (2015): 709–19. For a primer on the tau protein, the genetics of Alzheimer's, see also "A Primer on Alzheimer's Disease and the Brain" at https://www .nia.nih.gov/alzheimers/publication/2011-2012-alzheimers-disease-progress-report /primer-alzheimers-disease-and.

13. V. K. Ramanan et al., "GWAS of Longitudinal Amyloid Accumulation on 18F-florbetapir PET in Alzheimer's Disease Implicates Microglial Activation Gene IL1RAP," *Brain* 138 (2015): 3076–88.

14. L. M. McConnell et al., "Genetic Testing and Alzheimer's Disease: Recommendations of the Stanford Program in Genomics, Ethics, and Society," *Genetic Testing* 3 (1999): 3–12.

15. Public Health Genetics Unit, "Alzheimer's Disease"; J. S. Goldman and C. E. Hou, "Early-Onset Alzheimer's Disease: When Is Genetic Testing Appropriate?" *Alzheimer's Disease and Related Disorders* 18 (2004): 65–67.

16. C. M. McBride, "Personal Genomic Tests for Healthy Aging: Neither Feast nor Foul," *Generations* 39, no. 1 (2015): 41.

## Notes to Chapter 5

1. American Psychiatric Association, *Diagnostic and Statistical Manual of Mental Disorders,* 5th ed. (Washington, DC: American Psychiatric Association, 2013).

2. E. D. Caine and H. T. Grossman, "Neuropsychiatric Assessment," in *Handbook of Mental Health and Aging,* ed. J. E. Birren, R. Sloan, and G. D. Cohen (San Diego: Academic Press, 1992), 603–42.

3. H. I. Kaplan and B. J. Saddock, eds. *Synopsis of Psychiatry* (Baltimore: Williams and Wilkins, 1994).

4. Caine and Grossman, "Neuropsychiatric Assessment"; Kaplan and Saddock, *Synopsis of Psychiatry.*

5. V. Ladislav et al., "Sundowning and Circadian Rhythms in Alzheimer's Disease," *American Journal of Psychiatry* 158 (2001): 704–11.

6. A. Satlin et al., "Bright Light Treatment of Behavioral and Sleep Disturbances in Patients with Alzheimer's Disease," *American Journal of Psychiatry* 149 (1992): 1028–32.

7. E. H. Liston, "Diagnosis and Management of Delirium in the Elderly Patient," *Psychiatric Annals* 14 (1984): 117.

8. V. C. Hachinski, "Differential Diagnosis of Alzheimer's Dementia: Multi-Infarct Dementia," in *Alzheimer's Disease: The Standard Reference,* ed. B. Reisberg (New York: Free Press, 1983), 188–92.

9. J. R. Youngjohn and T. H. Crook, "Dementia," in *The Practical Handbook of Clinical Gerontology,* ed. L. L. Carstensen, B. A. Edelstein, and L. Dornbrand (Thousand Oaks, CA: Sage, 1996), 76–106.

10. J. L. Cummings and D. F. Benson, *Dementia: A Clinical Approach,* 2nd ed. (Boston: Butterworth-Heinemann, 1992).

## Note to Chapter 6

1. M. Crisby, L. A. Carlson, and B. Winblad, "Statins in the Prevention and Treatment of Alzheimer's Disease," *Alzheimer Disease and Associated Disorders* 16 (2002): 131–36.

## Notes to Chapter 7

1. A. La Rue, J. Yang, and S. Osato "Neuropsychological Assessment," in *Handbook of Mental Health and Aging,* ed. J. E. Birren, R. B. Sloan, and G. D. Cohen (San Diego: Academic Press, 1992), 643–70. See also B. Reisberg, "Alzheimer's Disease," in *Comprehensive Review of Geriatric Psychiatry—II,* ed. ed. J. Sadavoy et al. (Washington, DC: American Psychiatric Press, 1996), 401–58.

2. H. I. Kaplan and B. J. Saddock, eds. *Synopsis of Psychiatry* (Baltimore: Williams and Wilkins, 1994).

3. S. K. Inouye et al., "Clarifying Confusion: The Confusion Assessment Method. A New Method for Detection of Delirium." *Annals of Internal Medicine* 113 (1990): 941–48.

4. S. H. Tariq, "Comparison of the Saint Louis University Mental Status Examination and the Mini-Mental State Examination for Detecting Dementia and Mild Neurocognitive Disorder: A Pilot Study," *American Journal of Geriatric Psychiatry* 14 (2006): 900–910. See also Z. S. Nasreddine et al., "The Montreal Cognitive Assessment, MoCA: A Brief Screening Tool for Mild Cognitive Impairment," *Journal of the American Geriatric Society* 53, no. 4 (2005): 695–99.

5. Z. S. Nasreddine et al., "The Montreal Cognitive Assessment, MoCA." The MoCA is freely available at http://www.mocatest.org and can be reproduced.

6. M. Critchley, "The Parietal Lobes," (New York: Hafner Publishing Company, 1953, reprinted 1966). See also, K. I. Shulman, R. Shedletsky, and I. L. Silver, "The Challenge of Time: Clock-Drawing and Cognitive Functioning in the Elderly," *International Journal of Geriatric Psychiatry* 1 (1986): 135–40.

7. H. Buschke et al., "Screening for Dementia with the Memory Impairment Screen," *Neurology* 52 (1999): 231–38.

8. The screening item shown is taken from G. Blessed, B. Tomlinson, and M. Roth. "The Association Between Quantitative Measures of Dementia and of Senile Change in the Cerebral Grey Matter of Elderly Subjects," *British Journal of Psychiatry* 114 (1968): 797–811.

9. S. Kilada et al., "Brief Screening Tests for the Diagnosis of Dementia: Comparison with the Mini-Mental State Exam," *Alzheimer Disease and Associated Disorders* 19 (2005): 8–16.

10. Psychological Assessment Resources, *The Dementia Rating Scale* (Odessa, FL: Psychological Assessment Resources, 2001); W. G. Rosen, R. C. Mohs, and K. L. Davis, "A New Rating Scale for Alzheimer's Disease," *American Journal of Psychiatry* 141 (1984): 1356–64. The instrument has been revised and is now called the *Dementia Rating Scale—2*.

11. D. Wechsler, *Wechsler Memory Scale—III, Manual* (San Antonio, TX: The Psychological Corporation, 1997).

12. A. J. Gibson and D. C. Kendrick, *The Kendrick Cognitive Tests for the Elderly* (Windsor, Berks, UK: NFER-Nelson, 1982).

13. E. F. Kaplan, H. Goodglass, and S. Weintraub, *The Boston Naming Test,* 2nd ed. (Philadelphia: Lea and Febiger, 1983).

14. R. K. Heaton et al., *Wisconsin Card Sorting Test Manual,* revised and expanded (Odessa, FL: Psychological Assessment Resources, 1993).

15. D. Wechsler, *Wechsler Adult Intelligence Scale—III* (San Antonio, TX: The Psychological Corporation, 1997).

16. For a compilation of psychological tests commonly used with the elderly, see A. Burns, B. Lawlor, and S. Craig, *Assessment Scales in Old Age Psychiatry* (London: Martin Dunitz, 1999).

17. L. Velayudhan, "Smell Identification Function and Alzheimer's Disease: a Selective Review," *Current Opinion in Psychiatry* 28, no. 2 (2015): 173–79. See also T. Field, "Smell and Taste Dysfunction as Early Markers for Neurodegenerative and Neuropsychiatric Diseases," *Journal of Alzheimers Disease & Parkinsonism* 2015 (2015). See also D. P. Devanand et al., "Olfactory Deficits in Patients with Mild Cognitive Impairment Predict Alzheimer's Disease at Follow-Up," *American Journal of Psychiatry* 157 (2000): 1399–1405.

## Notes to Chapter 8

1. Tom Tuttle (personal communication, November 2003).

2. B. Reisberg et al., "The Global Deterioration Scale for Assessment of Primary Degenerative Dementia," *American Journal of Psychiatry* 139 (1982): 1136–39.

3. E. Cohen, *The House on Beartown Road: A Memoir of Learning and Forgetting* (New York: Random House, 2003).

4. B. Brock et al., *Reality Comprehension Clock Test* (Toledo, OH: Communication Art, 1999); R. Olsson, R. Kucharewski, and H. Eichner, "The Reality Comprehension Clock Test: A Validity Analysis," *Expanding Horizons in Therapeutic Recreation* 19 (2001): 128–32.

5. B. J. Kemp and J. M. Mitchell, "Functional Assessment in Geriatric Mental Health," in *Handbook of Mental Health and Aging,* ed. J. E. Birren, R. B. Sloan, and G. D. Cohen (San Diego: Academic Press, 1992), 671–97.

6. D. Loewenstein et al., "A New Scale for the Functional Status in Alzheimer's and Related Disorders," *Journal of Gerontology* 44 (1989): 114–21.

7. J. D'Andrea et al., "The Community Competence Scale—Short Form: A Competency-Based Measure for Determining Residential Placement of Geriatric Patients," *Clinical Gerontologist* 4 (1991): 3–10.

8. S. Teunisse and M. M. A. Derix, "The Interview for Deterioration in Daily Living Activities in Dementia: Agreement Between Primary and Secondary Caregivers," *International Psychogeriatrics* 9 (1997): 155–62.

## Notes to Chapter 9

1. T. Grisso, "Clinical Assessments of Legal Competence of Older Adults," in *Neuropsychological Assessment of Dementia and Depression in Older Adults,* ed. M. Storandt and G. R. Vandenbos (Washington, DC: American Psychological Association, 1994), 119–40.

2. For a general discussion of the topic, see, for example, M. B. Kapp, "Assessment of Competence to Make Medical Decisions," in *The Practical Handbook of Clinical Gerontology,* ed. L. L. Carstensen, B. A. Edelstein, and L. Dornbrand (Thousand Oaks, CA: Sage, 1996), 174–87.

3. T. Grisso and P. S. Appelbaum. *Assessing Competence to Consent to Treatment: A Guide for Physicians and Other Health Care Professionals* (New York: Oxford University Press, 1998).

4. L. B. Lisis and S. Barinaga-Burch, "National Study of Guardianship Systems: Summary of Findings and Recommendations," *Clearinghouse Review* 29 (1995): 643.

5. L. Ganzini et al., "Ten Myths about Decision-Making Capacity," *Journal of the American Medical Directors Association* 6 (2005): S100–S104.

6. N. Karp and E. F. Wood, "Guardianship Monitoring: A National Survey of Court Practices," *Stetson Law Review* 37 (2007): 143.

7. American Bar Association Commission on Law and Aging and American Psychological Association Assessment of Capacity in Older Adults Project Working Group, *Assessment of Older Adults with Diminished Capacity: A Handbook for Psychologists* (American Bar Association and American Psychological Association, 2008), www.apa.org/pi/aging/capacity_psychologist_handbook.pdf; American Bar Association Commission on Law and Aging, American Psychological Association, and National College of Probate Judges, *Judicial Determination of Capacity of Older Adults in Guardianship Proceedings: A Handbook for Judges* (American Bar

Association and American Psychological Association, 2006), www.abanet.org/aging /docs/judges_book_5-24.pdf.

8. D. Iverson et al., "Practice Parameter Update: Evaluation and Management of Driving Risk in Dementia: Report of the Quality Standards Subcommittee of the American Academy of Neurology," *Neurology* 74 (2010): 1316–24.

9. To learn more about the Uniform Probate Code, visit Cornell University Law School's Legal Information Institute at www.law.cornell.edu/uniform/probate.

10. Grisso and Appelbaum, *Assessing Competence to Consent to Treatment.*

11. J. Moye, "Guardianship and Conservatorship," in *Evaluating Competencies: Forensic Assessments and Instruments,* 2nd ed., ed. T. Grisso (New York: Springer, 2003), 309–89. See also J. Moye, D. C. Marson, and B. Edelstein, "Assessment of Capacity in an Aging Society," *American Psychologist* 68, no. 3 (2013): 158–71.

12. L. A. Frolik, "Promoting Judicial Acceptance and Use of Limited Guardianship," *Stetson Law Review* 31 (2002): 737.

13. Ibid.

14. Uniform Probate Code § 5-102 (amended 2010).

15. J. Moye, "Guardianship and Conservatorship."

16. J. S. Janofsky et al., "The Hopkins Competency Assessment Test: A Brief Method for Evaluating Patients' Capacity to Give Informed Consent," *Hospital and Community Psychiatry* 43 (1992): 132–35.

17. T. Grisso et al., "The MacCAT-T: A Clinical Tool to Assess Patients' Capacities to Make Treatment Decisions," *Psychiatric Services* 48, no. 11 (1997): 1415–19. See also J. Moye, M. J. Karel, B. Edelstein, B. Hicken, J. C. Armesto, and R. J. Gurrera, "Assessment of Capacity to Consent to Treatment" *Clinical Gerontologist* 31 (2007): 37–66.

## Notes to Chapter 10

1. U.S. Department of Health and Human Services, *Mental Health: A Report of the Surgeon General* (Rockville, MD: U.S. Department of Health and Human Services, 1999). Available online at https://profiles.nlm.nih.gov/ps/access/NNBBHS.pdf.

2. R. Wolfe, J. Morrow, and B. L. Fredrickson, "Mood Disorders in Older Adults," in *The Practical Handbook of Clinical Gerontology,* ed. L. L. Carstensen, B. A. Edelstein, and L. Dornbrand (Thousand Oaks, CA: Sage, 1996), 274–303.

3. J. J. Locascio, J. H. Growdon, and S. Corkin, "Cognitive Test Performance in Detecting, Staging, and Tracking Alzheimer's Disease," *Archives of Neurology* 52 (1995): 1087–99.

4. W. D. Taylor et al., "The Vascular Depression Hypothesis: Mechanisms Linking Vascular Disease with Depression," *Molecular Psychiatry* 18, no. 9 (2013): 963–74.

See also K. R. Rama Krishnan, "Vascular Disease and Depression," *Audio Digest Psychiatry* 34, no. 1 (January 7, 2005); B. T. Mast, B. Yochim, S. E. MacNeil, and P. A. Lichtenberg. "Risk Factors for Geriatric Depression: The Importance of Executive Functioning within the Vascular Depression Hypothesis," *Journals of Gerontology, Series A: Biological Sciences and Medical Sciences* 59 (2004): 1290–94.

5. American Psychiatric Association, *Diagnostic and Statistical Manual of Mental Disorders,* 5th ed. (Washington, DC: American Psychiatric Association, 2013).

6. J. I. Sheikh and J. A. Yesavage, "Geriatric Depression Scale (GDS): Recent Evidence and Development of a Shorter Version," in *Clinical Gerontology: A Guide to Assessment and Intervention,* ed. T. L. Brink (New York: Haworth Press, 1988), 165–73.

7. C. G. Lyketsos, "Current Issues in Dementia Care," *Audio Digest Psychiatry* 33, no. 18 (21 September 2004).

8. G. S. Alexopoulos et al., "Cornell Scale for Depression in Dementia," *Biological Psychiatry* 23 no. 3 (1988): 271–84.

9. Wolfe, Morrow, and Fredrickson, "Mood Disorders in Older Adults."

10. Ibid.; M. A. Raskind and E. R. Peskind, "Alzheimer's Disease and Other Dementing Disorders," in *Handbook of Mental Health and Aging,* ed. J. E. Birren, R. B. Sloan, and G. D. Cohen (San Diego: Academic Press, 1992), 477–513.

11. A. La Rue, J. Yang, and S. Osato, "Neuropsychological Assessment," in *Handbook of Mental Health and Aging,* ed. J. E. Birren, R. B. Sloan, and G. D. Cohen (San Diego: Academic Press, 1992), 643–70.

12. A. W. Kaszniak and G. D. Christenson, "Differential Diagnosis of Dementia and Depression," in *Neuropsychological Assessment of Dementia and Depression in Older Adults,* ed. M. Storandt and G. R. Vandenbos (Washington, DC: American Psychological Association, 1998), 81–118.

## Notes to Chapter 11

1. B. C. Jost and G. T. Grossberg, "The Evolution of Psychiatric Symptoms in Alzheimer's Disease: A Natural History Study," *Journal of the American Geriatrics Society* 44, no. 9 (1996): 1078–81.

2. G. W. Strahan, *Mental Illness in Nursing Homes* (Hyattsville, MD: U.S. Department of Health and Human Services, 1985). Also see G. W. Strahan, *An Overview of Nursing Homes and Their Current Residents: Data from the 1995 National Nursing Home Survey* (Hyattsville, MD: U.S. Department of Health and Human Services, 1995).

3. U.S. Department of Health and Human Services, *Mental Health: A Report of the Surgeon General* (Rockville, MD: U.S. Department of Health and Human Services,

1999). Available online at https://profiles.nlm.nih.gov/ps/access/NNBBHS.pdf.

4. G. Pearlson and P. Rabins, "The Late Onset Psychosis: Possible Risk Factors," *Psychiatric Clinics of North America* 11 (1988): 15–32.

5. U.S. Department of Health and Human Services, *Mental Health.*

6. J. Marengo and J. F. Westermeyer, "Schizophrenia and Delusional Disorder," in *The Practical Handbook of Clinical Gerontology,* ed. L. L. Carstensen, B. A. Edelstein, and L. Dornbrand (Thousand Oaks, CA: Sage, 1996), 255–73.

7. H. I. Kaplan and B. J. Saddock, eds., *Synopsis of Psychiatry* (Baltimore: Williams and Wilkins, 1994).

## Notes to Chapter 12

1. T. DeBaggio, *Losing My Mind: An Intimate Look at Life with Alzheimer's* (New York: Simon and Schuster Audio, 2002).

2. A. Qaseem et al., "Current Pharmacologic Treatment of Dementia: A Clinical Practice Guideline from the American College of Physicians and the American Academy of Family Physicians," *Annals of Internal Medicine* 148 (2008): 370–78.

3. N. R. Carlson, *Foundations of Physiological Psychology* (Needham, MA: Allyn & Bacon, 1995).

4. J. Bryant et al., "Clinical and Cost Effectiveness of Donepezil, Rivastigmine, and Galantamine for Alzheimer's Disease: A Rapid and Systematic Review," *Health Technology Assessment* 5 (2001): 1–137.

5. J. L. Cummings et al., "Guidelines for Managing Alzheimer's Disease: Part II, Treatment," *American Family Physician* 65 (2002): 2525–64.

6. Underwood, E. "Alzheimer's Amyloid Theory Gets Modest Boost," *Science* 349, (2015): 464–464.

7. M. G. Agadjanyan et al., "A Fresh Perspective from Immunologists and Vaccine Researchers: Active Vaccination Strategies to Prevent and Reverse Alzheimer's Disease," *Alzheimer's & Dementia* 11 (2015): 1246–59.

8. N. Relkin, "Clinical Trials of Intravenous Immunoglobulin for Alzheimer's Disease," *Journal of Clinical Immunology* 34, no. 1 (2014): 74–79.

9. K. Blennow and H. Zetterberg, "The Past and the Future of Alzheimer's Disease CSF Biomarkers: A Journey Toward Validated Biochemical Tests Covering the Whole Spectrum of Molecular Events," *Frontiers in Neuroscience* 9, http://dx.doi .org/10.3389/fnins.2015.00345

10. P. S. Aisen et al., "Effects of Rofecoxib or Naproxen vs. Placebo on Alzheimer Disease: A Randomly Controlled Trial," *Journal of the American Medical Association* 289 (2003): 2819–26.

11. M. Miguel-Álvarez, A. Santos-Lozano, F. Sanchis-Gomar, C. Fiuza-Luces, H.

Pareja-Galeano, N. Garatachea, and A. Lucia. "Non-steroidal Anti-inflammatory Drugs as a Treatment for Alzheimer's Disease: A Systematic Review and Meta-analysis of Treatment Effect," *Drugs & Aging* 32 (2015): 139–47.

12. P. Chakrabarty et al., "IL-10 Alters Immunoproteostasis in APP Mice, Increasing Plaque Burden and Worsening Cognitive Behavior," *Neuron* 85 (2015): 519–33.

13. L. Packer and C. Colman, *The Antioxidant Miracle: Your Complete Plan for Total Health* (New York: Wiley, 1999).

14. M. O. Grimm et al., "Vitamin E: Curse or Benefit in Alzheimer's Disease? A Systematic Investigation of the Impact of α-, γ- and δ-tocopherol on Aβ Generation and Degradation in Neuroblastoma Cells," *The Journal of Nutrition, Health & Aging* (2015): 1–9.

15. M. Naoi et al., "Modulation of Monoamine Oxidase (MAO) Expression in Neuropsychiatric Disorders: Genetic and Environmental Factors Involved in Type A MAO Expression," *Journal of Neural Transmission* (2015): 1–16. See also R. Mayeux and M. Sano, "Treatment of Alzheimer's Disease," *New England Journal of Medicine* 341 (1999): 1670–79.

16. R. P. Friedland, "Fish Consumption and the Risk of Alzheimer's Disease: It's Time to Make Dietary Recommendations," *Archives of Neurology* 60 (2003): 923–24.

17. M. A. Phillips et al., "No Effect of Omega-3 Fatty Acid Supplementation on Cognition and Mood in Individuals with Cognitive Impairment and Probable Alzheimer's Disease: A Randomised Controlled Trial," *International Journal of Molecular Sciences* 16, no. 10 (2015): 24600–24613. See also S. Wu et al., "Omega-3 Fatty Acids Intake and Risks of Dementia and Alzheimer's Disease: A Meta-analysis," *Neuroscience & Biobehavioral Reviews* 48 (2015): 1–9.

18. L. Shen and H. F. Ji, "Associations Between Homocysteine, Folic Acid, Vitamin B12 and Alzheimer's Disease: Insights from Meta-Analyses," *Journal of Alzheimer's Disease: JAD* (2015).

19. A. Storch et al., "Adult Human Bone Marrow-Derived Neural Stem Cells: A New Cell Source for Neurorestorative Strategies" (56th Annual Meeting of the Academy of Neurology, San Francisco, CA, April 30, 2004).

20. R. R. Ager et al., "Human Neural Stem Cells Improve Cognition and Promote Synaptic Growth in Two Complementary Transgenic Models of Alzheimer's Disease and Neuronal Loss," *Hippocampus* 25, no. 7 (2015): 813–26.

21. S. A. Shumaker et al., "Estrogen Plus Progestin and the Incidence of Dementia and Mild Cognitive Impairment in Postmenopausal Women: The Women's Health Initiative Memory Study—A Randomized Controlled Trial," *Journal of the American Medical Association* 289 (2003): 2651–62.

22. V. Burnham and J. Thornton, "Luteinizing Hormone as a Key Player in the Cognitive Decline of Alzheimer's Disease," *Hormones and Behavior* (2015). See also K. W. Webber et al., "Gender Differences in Alzheimer's Disease: The Role of Luteinizing Hormone in Disease Pathogenesis," *Alzheimer Disease and Associated Disorders* 19 (2005): 95–99.

23. R. Mayeux and M. Sano, "Treatment of Alzheimer's Disease," *New England Journal of Medicine* 341 (1999): 1670–79.

24. S. T. DeKosky et al., "Ginkgo Biloba for Prevention of Dementia: A Randomized Controlled Trial," *Journal of the American Medical Association* 300 (2008): 2253–62.

25. J. Zhang, "Effect of Metal Ions and EDTA on Catalase Activity-Potential in Alzheimer's Treatment," (meeting, AAAS, February 12–16, 2015). See also N. G. Milton, "The Role of Hydrogen Peroxide in the Aetiology of Alzheimer's Disease: Implications for Treatment," *Drugs and Aging* 21 (2004): 81–100.

26. See, for example, S. M. de la Monti and J. R. Wands, "Alzheimer's Disease Is Type 3 Diabetes: Evidence Reviewed," *Journal of Diabetes Science and Technology* 2 (2008): 1101–13. See also M. Barbagallo and L. G. Dominguez, "Type 2 Diabetes Mellitus and Alzheimer's Disease. *World Journal of Diabetes* 5 (2014): 889–93.

27. M. C. Morris et al., "MIND Diet Associated with Reduced Incidence of Alzheimer's Disease," *Alzheimer's Dementia* 11 (2015): 1007–14.

28. R. S. Turner et al., "A Randomized, Double-Blind, Placebo-Controlled Trial of Resveratrol for Alzheimer Disease," *Neurology* 85 (2015): 1383–91.

29. M. Meinzer et al., "Transcranial Direct Current Stimulation in Mild Cognitive Impairment: Behavioral Effects and Neural Mechanisms," *Alzheimer's & Dementia* 11 (2015): 1032–40.

30. E. B. Larson, et al., "Exercise is Associated with Reduced Risk for Incident Dementia among Persons 65 Years of Age and Older," *Annals of Internal Medicine* 144 (2006): 73–81.

31. R. McClure et al., "Inhalable Curcumin: Offering the Potential for Translation to Imaging and Treatment of Alzheimer's Disease," *Journal of Alzheimer's Disease* 44 (2015): 283–95.

32. C. Cao, "The Potential Therapeutic Effects of THC on Alzheimer's Disease," *Journal of Alzheimer's Disease* 42 (2014): 973–84. See also B. G. Ramírez et al., "Prevention of Alzheimer's Disease Pathology by Cannabinoids: Neuroprotection Mediated by Blockade of Microglial Activation," *Journal of Neuroscience* 25 (2014): 1904–13.

33. M. J. Kan et al., "Arginine Deprivation and Immune Suppression in a Mouse Model of Alzheimer's Disease," *Journal of Neuroscience* 35 (2015): 5969–82.

34. Y. A. Sulistio and K. Heese, "Proteomics in Traditional Chinese Medicine with an

Emphasis on Alzheimer's Disease," *Evidence-Based Complementary and Alternative Medicine* 2015 (2015). See also P. M. Kidd, "A Review of Nutrients and Botanicals in the Integrative Management of Cognitive Dysfunction," *Alternative Medicine* 3 (1999): 144–161. See also the September 2002 issue of *Life Extension Magazine* for abstract summaries of studies related to alternative medicines in the treatment of cognitive impairment.

35. R. A. Whitmer et al., "Obesity in Middle Age and Future Risk of Dementia: A 27-year Longitudinal Population Based Study," *British Medical Journal* 330 (2005): 1360.

36. J. T. Yu and L. Tan, "Lifestyle Changes Might Prevent Alzheimer's Disease," *Annals of Translational Medicine* 3, no. 15 (2015).

37. M. Boccia et al., "Neuroanatomy of Alzheimer's Disease and Late-Life Depression: A Coordinate-Based Meta-Analysis of MRI Studies," *Journal of Alzheimer's disease: JAD* (2015). See also F. Ezekiel et al., "Comparisons Between Global and Focal Brain Atrophy Rates in Normal Aging and Alzheimer Disease: Boundary Shift Integral versus Tracing of the Entorhinal Cortex and Hippocampus," *Alzheimer Disease and Associated Disorders* 18 (2004), 196–201.

38. A. Gupta and C. Iadecola, "Impaired Aβ Clearance: A Potential Link Between Atherosclerosis and Alzheimer's Disease," *Name: Frontiers in Aging Neuroscience* 7 (2015): 115. See also *American Journal of Pathology,* news release, 21 July 2005.

39. M. Gatz et al., "Potential Modifiable Risk Factors for Dementia: Evidence from Identical Twins" (Alzheimer's Association International Conference on Prevention of Dementia: Early Diagnosis and Intervention Program, Washington, DC, June 18–21, 2005).

40. C. Laske et al., "Innovative Diagnostic Tools for Early Detection of Alzheimer's Disease," *Alzheimer's & Dementia* 11 (2015): 561–78.

41. R. Borroni et al., "Peripheral Blood Abnormalities in Alzheimer's Disease: Evidence for Early Endothelial Dysfunction," *Alzheimer Disease and Associated Disorders* 16 (2002): 150–55.

42. M. D. Murray et al., "Preservation of Cognitive Function with Antihypertensive Medications," *Archives of Internal Medicine* 162 (2002): 2090–96.

43. H. L. Daneschvar et al., "Do Statins Prevent Alzheimer's Disease? A Narrative Review," *European Journal of Internal Medicine* 26, no. 9 (2015): 666–69; M. Crisby, L. A. Carlson, and B. Winblad, "Statins in the Prevention and Treatment of Alzheimer's Disease," *Alzheimer Disease and Associated Disorders* 16 (2002): 131–36; J. C. Morris, "Dementia Update 2005," *Alzheimer Disease and Associated Disorders* 19 (2005): 100–117.

44. J. L. Cummings et al., "Guidelines for Managing Alzheimer's Disease"; J. Schneider, "Geriatric Psychopharmacology," in *The Practical Handbook of Clinical*

*Gerontology,* ed. L. L. Carstensen, B. A. Edelstein, and L. Dornbrand (Thousand Oaks, CA: Sage, 1996), 481–542.

45. G. Fàzzari et al., "Maintenance ECT for the Treatment and Resolution of Agitation in Alzheimer's Dementia," *Journal of Psychopathology* 21 (2015): 159–160. See also L. Emsell et al., "How Do Age-Related White Matter Changes Such as MRI Hyperintensities and Amyloid Deposition Relate to ECT Outcome in Late Life Depression?" *European Psychiatry* 30 (2015): 135.

46. C. G. Lyketsos, "Current Issues in Dementia Care," *Audio Digest Psychiatry* 33, no. 18 (2004).

47. J. Kornfield, *Buddha's Little Instruction Book* (New York: Bantam, 1994).

## Notes to Chapter 13

1. M. L. Warner, *The Complete Guide to Alzheimer's-Proofing Your Home* (West Lafayette, IN: Purdue University Press, 2000). Also, the Alzheimer's Association has a program called "Safe Return" for protecting the safety of Alzheimer's sufferers who become lost outside the home. In this program, people with Alzheimer's are identified by an ID bracelet that they wear. This is a 24-hour nationwide network that can be contacted by calling toll-free (800) 272-3900.

2. V. Regnier and J. Pynoos, "Environmental Intervention for Cognitively Impaired Older Persons," in *Handbook of Mental Health and Aging,* ed. J. E. Birren, R. B. Sloan, and G. D. Cohen (San Diego: Academic Press, 1992), 763–92.

3. M. Bozich and S. Housley (unpublished manuscript, 1985), cited in B. H. Mulsant and J. Rosen, "Dementia (Alzheimer's Disease)," in *Handbook of Prescriptive Treatments for Adults,* ed. M. Hersen and R. T. Ammerman (New York: Plenum, 1994), 43.

## Notes to Chapter 14

1. Quoted in S. Giga, "Director's Corner," *Family and Children First News: A Newsletter of the Greene County [Ohio] Family and Children First Council,* n.d.

2. These two quotes were taken from a wonderful book by George Bouklas—G. Bouklas, *Psychotherapy with the Elderly: Becoming Methuselah's Echo* (New York: Aronson, 1997).

3. H. S. Sullivan, *The Interpersonal Theory of Psychiatry* (New York: Norton, 1953).

4. W. S. Sahakian, *Psychotherapy and Counseling: Techniques in Intervention* (Chicago, IL: Rand McNally, 1976).

5. M. D. Miller and R. L. Silberman, "Using Interpersonal Psychotherapy with Depressed Elders," in *A Guide to Psychotherapy and Aging,* ed. S. H. Zarit and B. G. Knight (Washington, DC: American Psychological Association Press, 1996), 83–99.

6. S. Freud, *An Outline of Psychoanalysis* (New York: Norton, 1949).

7. H. D. Lerner, "Psychodynamic Issues," in *Handbook of Clinical Geropsychology,* ed. M. Hersen and V. B. Van Hasselt (New York: Plenum, 1998), 29–50.

8. K. Sharoff, *Coping Skills for Managing Chronic and Terminal Illness* (New York: Springer, 2004).

9. L. W. Dupree and L. Schonfeld, "The Value of Behavioral Perspectives in Treating Older Adults," in *Handbook of Clinical Geropsychology,* M. Hersen and V. B. Van Hasselt (New York: Plenum, 1998), 51–70.

10. R. G. Logsdon and L. Teri, "The Pleasant Events Schedule—AD," *Gerontologist* 37 (1997): 40–45; R. G. Logsdon and L. Teri, "Identifying Pleasant Activities for Alzheimer's Patients: The Pleasant Events Schedule—AD," *Gerontologist* 31 (1991): 124–27.

11. A. S. Gurman and D. P. Kriskern, eds. *Handbook of Family Therapy,* vol. 2 (New York: Taylor and Francis, 1991).

12. Ibid.

13. S. H. Zarit, N. K. Orr, and J. M. Zarit, *The Hidden Victims of Alzheimer's Disease: Families under Stress* (New York: New York University Press, 1985); See also S. H. Zarit, K. E. Reever, and J. Bach-Peterson, "Relatives of the Impaired Elderly: Correlates of Feelings of Burden," *The Gerontologist* 20 (1980): 649–55; R. Petersen, ed. *Mayo Clinic on Alzheimer's Disease* (Rochester, MN: Mayo Clinic Health Information, 2002); L. Powell, *Alzheimer's Disease: A Guide for Families and Caregivers* (Cambridge, MA: Perseus, 2002).

14. K. E. Cherry and S. S. Simmons-D'Gerolamo, "Long-term Effectiveness of Spaced-retrieval Memory Training for Older Adults with Probable Alzheimer's Disease," *Experimental Aging Research* 31 (2005): 261–89.

15. M. Bourgeois et al., "Memory Aids as an Augmentative and Alternative Communication Strategy for Nursing Home Residents with Dementia," *Augmentative and Alternative Communication* 17 (2001): 196–210.

16. D. A. Snowdon, S. J. Kemper, and J. A. Mortimer, "Linguistic Ability in Early Life and Cognitive Function and Alzheimer's Disease in Late Life," *Journal of the American Medical Association* 275 (1996): 528–32; See also S. B. Chapman et al., "Discourse Changes in Early Alzheimer Disease, Mild Cognitive Impairment, and Normal Aging," *Alzheimer Disease and Associated Disorders* 16 (2002): 177–86.

## Notes to Chapter 15

1. G. E. Vaillant, *Aging Well: Surprising Guideposts to a Happier Life from the Landmark Harvard Study of Adult Development* (New York: Little, Brown and Company, 2002). See also J. Victoroff, *Saving Your Brain: The Revolutionary Way*

*to Boost Brain Power, Improve Memory, and Protect Yourself against Aging and Alzheimer's* (New York: Bantam Dell, 2002).

2. H. I. Zonneveld et al., "The Bidirectional Association Between Reduced Cerebral Blood Flow and Brain Atrophy in the General Population," *Journal of Cerebral Blood Flow & Metabolism* 35, no. 11 (2015): 1882–87. Earlier studies can be found in an article by T. Needels and T. Bilanow, "Power Up Your Brain," *Psychology Today,* August 2002, 44–51.

3. T. Archer and D. Garcia, "Physical Exercise Improves Cognition in Brain Disorders: Alzheimer's Disease," in *Diet and Exercise in Cognitive Function and Neurological Diseases,* (London: Wiley-Blackwell Publishing, 2015), 175–81. See also U.S. Department of Health and Human Services, "Dietary Guidelines for Americans," (Washington, DC: U.S. Department of Health and Human Services, 2005).

4. A Gupta and C. Iadecola, "Impaired Aβ Clearance: a Potential Link between Atherosclerosis and Alzheimer's Disease," *Name: Frontiers in Aging Neuroscience* 7 (2015): 115. See also M. Sjogren and K. Blennow, "The Link Between Cholesterol and Alzheimer's Disease," *World Journal of Biological Psychiatry* 6 (2005): 85–97.

5. M. C. Morris et al., "MIND Diet Associated with Reduced Incidence of Alzheimer's Disease," *Alzheimer's Dementia* 11 (2015): 1007–14. See also U.S. Department of Health and Human Services, "Dietary Guidelines for Americans."

6. E. Marcello, "Alzheimer's Disease and Modern Lifestyle: What is the Role of Stress?" *Journal of Neurochemistry* 134, no. 5 (2015): 795–98. See also T. Needels and T. Bilanow, "Power Up Your Brain," *Psychology Today,* August 2002, 44–51.

7. L. C. Katz and M. Rubin, *How to Keep Your Brain Alive: 83 Neurobic Exercises to Help Prevent Memory Loss and Increase Mental Fitness* (New York: Workman, 1999).

8. L. Buscaglia, *The Fall of Freddie the Leaf: A Story of Life for All Ages* (Thorofare, NJ: Slack, Inc., 1982).

9. *Reminisce: The Magazine That Brings Back the Good Times,* March/April 2002. Additional activities for the elderly can be found in *Creative Forecasting: A Monthly Periodical for Activity and Recreation Professionals* (Colorado Springs, CO: Creative Forecasting, Inc.); the publisher can be reached by calling (800) 373-0115.

10. Other mental and physical activities can be found in M. Engleman, *Aerobics of the Mind* (State College, PA: Venture, 1996); M. Hook, *Gentle Exercises and Movement for Frail People* (Plainview, NY: Wellness Reproductions, n.d.); and P. Nekola, *An Alzheimer's Guide: Activities and Issues for People Who Care* (Waukesha, WI: Applewood Ink, 2002).

11. Special thanks to Jackie Davis, MT-BC (Personal communication, August 2002) for providing these exercises.

## Note to Appendix B

1. The "6 R's" (Restrict, Reassess, Reconsider, Rechannel, Reassure, and Review) used to organize this section were developed by L. N. Mace and P. V. Rabins, *The 36 Hour Day* (Baltimore: Johns Hopkins University Press, 1996).

## Note to Appendix C

1. U.S. Department of Health and Human Services, *Mental Health: A Report of the Surgeon General* (Rockville, MD: U.S. Department of Health and Human Services, 1999). Available online at https://profiles.nlm.nih.gov/ps/access/NNBBHS.pdf.

# Bibliography

Agadjanyan, M. G., N. Petrovsky, and A. Ghochikyan. "A Fresh Perspective from Immunologists and Vaccine Researchers: Active Vaccination Strategies to Prevent and Reverse Alzheimer's Disease." *Alzheimer's & Dementia* 11 (2015): 1246–59. http://dx.doi.org/10.1016/j.jalz.2015.06.1884.

Ager, R. R., J. L. Davis, A. Agazaryan, F. Benavente, W. W. Poon, F. M. LaFerla, and M. Blurton-Jones. "Human Neural Stem Cells Improve Cognition and Promote Synaptic Growth in Two Complementary Transgenic Models of Alzheimer's Disease and Neuronal Loss." *Hippocampus* 25, no. 7 (2015): 813–26. http://dx.doi.org/10.1002/hipo.22405.

Aisen, P. S., K. A. Schafer, M. Grundman, E. Pfeiffer, M. Sano, K. L. Davis, M. R. Farlow, S. Jin, R. G. Thomas, and L. J. Thal. "Effects of Rofecoxib or Naproxen vs. Placebo on Alzheimer Disease: A Randomly Controlled Trial." *Journal of the American Medical Association* 289 (2003): 2819–26. http://dx.doi.org/10.1001/jama.289.21.2819.

Alexopoulos, G. S., R. C. Abrams, R. C. Young, and C. A. Shamoian. "Cornell Scale of Depression in Dementia." *Biological Psychiatry* 23 (1998): 271–84. http://dx.doi.org/10.1016/0006-3223(88)90038-8.

Alzheimer's Association. "Alzheimer's Disease Facts and Figures." *Alzheimer's & Dementia: The Journal of the Alzheimer's Association* 11, no. 3 (2015): 332.

American Bar Association Commission on Law and Aging and American Psychological Association Assessment of Capacity in Older Adults Project Working Group. *Assessment of Older Adults with Diminished Capacity: A Handbook for Psychologists.* American Bar Association and American Psychological Association, 2008. www.apa.org/pi/aging/capacity_psychologist_handbook.pdf.

American Bar Association Commission on Law and Aging, American Psychological Association, and National College of Probate Judges. *Judicial Determination of Capacity of Older Adults in Guardianship Proceedings: A Handbook for Judges.*

American Bar Association and American Psychological Association, 2006. https://www.apa.org/pi/aging/resources/guides/judges-diminished.pdf.

American Psychiatric Association. *Diagnostic and Statistical Manual of Mental Disorders.* 4th ed. Washington, DC: American Psychiatric Association, 1994.

American Psychiatric Association. *Diagnostic and Statistical Manual of Mental Disorders.* 5th ed. Washington, DC: American Psychiatric Association, 2013.

American Psychological Association. "Reports of the Association: Guidelines for the Evaluation of Dementia and Age-Related Cognitive Decline." *American Psychologist* 53 (1998): 1298–1303. http://dx.doi.org/10.1037/0003-066X.53.12.1298.

Archer, T., and D. Garcia. "Physical Exercise Improves Cognition in Brain Disorders: Alzheimer's Disease." In *Diet and Exercise in Cognitive Function and Neurological Diseases,* edited by Akhlaq A. Farooqui and Tahira Farooqui, 175–82. London: Wiley-Blackwell Publishing, 2015. http://dx.doi.org/10.1002/9781118840634.ch16.

Barbagallo, M., and L. G. Dominguez. "Type 2 Diabetes Mellitus and Alzheimer's Disease." *World Journal of Diabetes* 5 (2014): 889–93. http://dx.doi.org/10.4239/wjd.v5.i6.889.

Bayda, E. *Being Zen.* Boston: Shambhala, 2002.

Bédard, M., D. W. Molloy, L. Squire, S. Dubois, J. A. Lever, and M. O'Donnell. "The Zarit Burden Interview a New Short Version and Screening Version." *The Gerontologist* 41, no. 5 (2001): 652–57. http://dx.doi.org/10.1093/geront/41.5.652.

Blennow, K., and H. Zetterberg. "The Past and the Future of Alzheimer's Disease CSF Biomarkers: A Journey toward Validated Biochemical Tests Covering the Whole Spectrum of Molecular Events." *Frontiers in Neuroscience* 9 (2015). http://dx.doi.org/10.3389/fnins.2015.00345.

Blessed G., B. Tomlinson, and M. Roth. "The Association Between Quantitative Measures of Dementia and of Senile Change in the Cerebral Grey Matter of Elderly Subjects." *British Journal of Psychiatry* 114 (1968): 797–811. http://dx.doi.org/10.1192/bjp.114.512.797.

Bouklas, G. *Psychotherapy with the Elderly: Becoming Methuselah's Echo.* New York: Jason Aronson, 1997.

Bourgeois, M., K. Djkstra, L. Burgio, and R. Allen-Burge. "Memory Aids as an Augmentative and Alternative Communication Strategy for Nursing Home Residents with Dementia." *Augmentative and Alternative Communication* 17 (2001): 196–210. http://dx.doi.org/10.1080/aac.17.3.196.210.

Breitner, J. C. "Clinical Genetics and Genetic Counseling in Alzheimer Disease." *Annals of Internal Medicine* 115 (1991): 601–6. http://dx.doi.org/10.7326/0003-4819-601.

Brock, B., L. Cousino, R. Olsson, P. Rostetter, R. Kucharewski, and L. Buchele. *Reality Comprehension Clock Test.* Toledo, OH: Communication Art, 1999.

Bryant, J., A. Clegg, T. Nicholson, L. McIntyre, S. DeBroe, K. Gerard, and N. Waugh. "Clinical and Cost Effectiveness of Donepezil, Rivastigmine, and Galantamine for Alzheimer's Disease—A Rapid and Systematic Review." *Health Technology Assessment* 5 (2001): 1–137. http://dx.doi.org/10.3310/hta5010.

Burns, A., B. Lawlor, and S. Craig. *Assessment Scales in Old Age Psychiatry.* London: Martin Dunitz, 1999.

Buscaglia, L. *The Fall of Freddie the Leaf: A Story of Life for All Ages.* Thorofare, NJ: Slack, Inc., 1982.

Buschke, H., G. Kuslansky, M. Katz, W. F. Stewart, M. J. Sliwinski, H. M. Eckholdt, and R. B. Lipton. "Screening for Dementia with the Memory Impairment Screen." *Neurology* 52 (1999): 231–38. http://dx.doi.org/10.1212/WNL.52.2.231.

Caine, E. D., and H. T. Grossman. "Neuropsychiatric Assessment." In *Handbook of Mental Health and Aging,* edited by J. E. Birren, R. B. Sloan, and G. D. Cohen, 603–42. San Diego: Academic Press, 1992. http://dx.doi.org/10.1016/B978-0-12-101277-9.50026-7.

Callahan, C. M., H. C. Hendrie, and W. M. Tierney. "Documentation and Evaluation of Cognitive Impairment in Elderly Primary Care Patients." *Annals of Internal Medicine* 122 (1995): 422–429. http://dx.doi.org/10.7326/0003-4819-122-6-199503150-00004.

Cao, C., Y. Li, H. Liu, G. Bai, J. Mayl, X. Lin, K. Sutherland, N. Nabare, and J. Cai. "The Potential Therapeutic Effects of THC on Alzheimer's Disease." *Journal of Alzheimer's Disease* 42 (2014): 973–84.

Carlson, N. R. *Foundations of Physiological Psychology.* Needham, MA: Allyn & Bacon, 1995.

Carpenter, B. D., C. Xiong, E. K. Porensky, M. M. Lee, P. J. Brown, M. Coats, D. Johnson, and J. C. Morris. "Reaction to a Dementia Diagnosis in Individuals with Alzheimer's Disease and Mild Cognitive Impairment." *Journal of the American Geriatrics Society* 56 (2008): 405–12. http://dx.doi.org/10.1111/j.1532-5415.2007.01600.x.

Chakrabarty, P., A. Li, C. Ceballos-Diaz, J. A. Eddy, C. C. Funk, B. Moore et al. "IL-10 Alters Immunoproteostasis in APP Mice, Increasing Plaque Burden and Worsening Cognitive Behavior." *Neuron* 85, no. 3 (2015): 519–33. http://dx.doi.org/10.1016/j .neuron.2014.11.020.

Chapman, S. B., J. Zientz, M. Weiner, R. Rosenberg, W. Frawley, and M. H. Burns. "Discourse Changes in Early Alzheimer Disease, Mild Cognitive Impairment, and Normal Aging." *Alzheimer Disease & Associated Disorders* 16, no. 3 (2002): 177–86. http://dx.doi.org/10.1097/00002093-200207000-00008.

Chen, J. C., S. Borson, and J. M. Scanlan. "Stage-Specific Prevalence of Behavioral Symptoms in Alzheimer's Disease in a Multi-ethnic Sample." *American Journal of Geriatric Psychiatry* 8 (2000): 123–33. http://dx.doi.org/10.1097/00019442-200005000 -00007.

Cherry, K. E., and S. S. Simmons-D'Gerolamo. "Long-Term Effectiveness of Spaced-Retrieval Memory Training for Older Adults with Probable Alzheimer's Disease." *Experimental Aging Research* 31 (2005): 261–89. http://dx.doi.org/10.1080/03610730590948186.

Chu, J., J. G. Li, Y. B. Joshi, P. F. Giannopoulos, N. E. Hoffman, M. Madesh, and D. Praticò. "Gamma Secretase-Activating Protein Is a Substrate for Caspase-3: Implications for Alzheimer's Disease." *Biological Psychiatry* 77, no. 8 (2015): 720–28. http://dx.doi .org/10.1016/j.biopsych.2014.06.003.

Coffey, C. E., J. A. Saxton, G. Ratcliff, R. N. Bryan, and J. F. Lucke. "Relation of Education to Brain Size in Normal Aging: Implications for the Reserve Hypothesis." *Neurology* 53 (1999): 189–96. http://dx.doi.org/10.1212/WNL.53.1.189.

Cohen, E. *The House on Beartown Road: A Memoir of Learning and Forgetting.* New York: Random House, 2003.

Cowles, C. M., ed. *2001 Nursing Home Statistical Yearbook.* Montgomery Village, MD: Cowles Research Group, 2002.

Crisby, M., L. A. Carlson, and B. Winblad. "Statins in the Prevention and Treatment of Alzheimer's Disease." *Alzheimer Disease and Associated Disorders* 16 (2002): 131–36. http://dx.doi.org/10.1097/00002093-200207000-00001.

Cummings, J. L. "Dementia and Depression: An Evolving Enigma." *Journal of Neuropsychiatry and Clinical Neurosciences* 1 (1989): 236–42. http://dx.doi.org/10.1176 /jnp.1.3.236.

Cummings, J. L., and D. F. Benson. *Dementia: A Clinical Approach.* 2nd ed. Boston: Butterworth-Heinemann, 1992.

Cummings, J. L., and D. V. Jeste. "Alzheimer's Disease and Its Management in the Year 2010." *Psychiatric Services* 50 (1999): 1173–77. http://dx.doi.org/10.1176/ps.50.9.1173.

Cummings, J. L., J. C. Frank, D. Cherry, N. D. Kohatsu, B. Kemp, L. Hewett, and B. Mittman. "Guidelines for Managing Alzheimer's Disease: Part II. Treatment." *American Family Physician* 65 (2002): 2525–34.

D'Andrea, J., M. A. Goldberg, H. R. Searight, F. Gilner, and B. Katz. "The Community Competence Scale—Short Form: A Competency-Based Measure for Determining Residential Placement of Geriatric Patients." *Clinical Gerontologist* 4 (1991): 3–10. http://dx.doi.org/10.1300/J018v10n04_02.

Daneschvar, H. L., M. D. Aronson, and G. W. Smetana. "Do Statins Prevent Alzheimer's Disease? A Narrative Review." *European Journal of Internal Medicine* 26, no. 9 (2015): 666–69. http://dx.doi.org/10.1016/j.ejim.2015.08.012.

De la Monti, S. M., and J. R. Wands. "Alzheimer's Disease Is Type 3 Diabetes—Evidence Reviewed." *Journal of Diabetes Science and Technology* 2 (2008): 1101–13. http:// dx.doi.org/10.1177/193229680800200619.

DeBaggio, T. *Losing My Mind: An Intimate Look at Life with Alzheimer's.* New York: Simon & Schuster Audio, 2002.

DeKosky, S. T., J. D. Williamson, A. L. Fitzpatrick, R. A. Kronmal, D. G. Ives, J. A. Saxton et al. "Ginkgo Biloba for Prevention of Dementia: A Randomized Controlled

Trial." *Journal of the American Medical Association* 300 (2008): 2253–62. http://dx.doi .org/10.1001/jama.2008.683.

Devanand, D. P., K. S. Michaels-Marston, X. Liu, G. H. Pelton, M. Padilla, K. Marder, K. Bell, Y. Stern, and R. Mayeux. "Olfactory Deficits in Patients with Mild Cognitive Impairment Predict Alzheimer's Disease at Follow-Up." *American Journal of Psychiatry* 157 (2000): 1399–1405. http://dx.doi.org/10.1176/appi.ajp.157.9.1399.

Duara, R., W. W. Barker, R. Lopez-Alberola, D. A. Loewenstein, L. B. Grau, D. Gilchrist, S. Sevush, and S. St. George-Hyslop. "Alzheimer's Disease: Interaction of Apolipoprotein E Genotype, Family History of Dementia, Gender, Education, Ethnicity, and Age of Onset." *Neurology* 46 (1996): 1575–79. http://dx.doi.org/10.1212/WNL.46.6.1575.

Dupree, L. W., and L. Schonfeld. "The Value of Behavioral Perspectives in Treating Older Adults." In *Handbook of Clinical Geropsychology,* edited by M. Hersen and V. B. Van Hasselt, 51–70. New York: Plenum, 1998. http://dx.doi.org/10.1007/978-1 -4899-0130-9_4.

Emery, V. O. B. *Pseudodementia: A Theoretical and Empirical Discussion.* Cleveland, OH: Western Reserve Geriatric Education Center, 1988.

Emsell, L., F. Bouckaert, F. L. De Winter, J. Obbels, A. Dols, M. Stek, P. Sienert, S. Sunaert, and M. Vandenbulcke. "How Do Age-Related White Matter Changes Such as MRI Hyperintensities and Amyloid Deposition Relate to ECT Outcome in Late Life Depression?" *European Psychiatry* 30 (2015): 135. http://dx.doi.org/10.1016 /S0924-9338(15)31838-1.

Engleman, M. *Aerobics of the Mind.* State College, PA: Venture, 1996.

Fàzzari, G., C. Marangoni, and O. Benzoni. "Maintenance ECT for the Treatment and Resolution of Agitation in Alzheimer's Dementia." *Journal of Psychopathology* 21 (2015): 159–60.

Field, T. "Smell and Taste Dysfunction as Early Markers for Neurodegenerative and Neuropsychiatric Diseases." *Journal of Alzheimers Disease & Parkinsonism* 5 (2015): 186. http://dx.doi.org/10.4172/2161-0460.1000186.

Foley, J. M., and A. L. Heck. "Neurocognitive Disorders in Aging: A Primer on DSM-5 Changes and Framework for Application to Practice." *Clinical Gerontologist* 37, no. 4 (2014): 317–46. http://dx.doi.org/10.1080/07317115.2014.907595.

Folstein, M. F., S. Folstein, and P. R. McHugh. "The Mini-Mental State: A Practical Method for Grading the Cognitive State of Patients for the Clinician." *Journal of Psychiatric Research* 12 (1975): 189. http://dx.doi.org/10.1016/0022-3956(75)90026-6.

Freud, S. *An Outline of Psychoanalysis.* New York: Norton, 1949.

Frolik, L. A. "Promoting Judicial Acceptance and Use of Limited Guardianship." *Stetson Law Review* 31 (2002): 735–55.

Ganzini, L., L. Volicer, W. Nelson, E. Fox, and A. Derse. "Ten Myths about Decision-Making

Capacity." *Journal of the American Medical Directors Association* 6 (2005): S100–S104. http://dx.doi.org/10.1016/j.jamda.2005.03.021.

Gatz, M., C. A. Reynolds, L. Fratiglioni, B. Johansson, J. A. Mortimer, S. Berg, A. Fiske, and N. L. Pedersen. "Role of Genes and Environments for Explaining Alzheimer Disease." *Archives of General Psychiatry* 63, no. 2 (2006): 168–74. http://dx.doi.org/10.1001/archpsyc.63.2.168.

Gibson, A. J., and D. C. Kendrick. *The Kendrick Cognitive Tests for the Elderly.* Winsor, Berks, UK: NFER-Nelson, 1982.

Golden, C. J., and A. Chronopolous. "Dementia." *Handbook of Clinical Geropsychology,* edited by M. Hersen and V. B. Van Hasselt, 113–45. New York: Plenum, 1998. http://dx.doi.org/10.1007/978-1-4899-0130-9_7.

Goldman, J. S., and C. E. Hou. "Early-onset Alzheimer's Disease: When Is Genetic Testing Appropriate?" *Alzheimer's Disease and Related Disorders* 18 (2004): 65–67. http://dx.doi.org/10.1097/01.wad.0000126616.77653.71.

Grimm, M. O., C. P. Stahlmann, J. Mett, V. J. Haupenthal, V. C. Zimmer, J. Lehmann, B. Hundsdörfer, K. Endres, H. S. Grimm, and T. Hartmann. "Vitamin E: Curse or Benefit in Alzheimer's Disease? A Systematic Investigation of the Impact of α-, γ-and δ-tocopherol on Aβ Generation and Degradation in Neuroblastoma Cells." *The Journal of Nutrition, Health & Aging* 19, no. 6 (2015): 646–56. http://dx.doi.org/10.1007/s12603-015-0506-z.

Grisso, T. "Clinical Assessments of Legal Competence of Older Adults." In *Neuropsychological Assessment of Dementia and Depression in Older Adults,* edited by M. Storandt and G. R. Vandenbos, 119–40. Washington, DC: American Psychological Association, 1994. http://dx.doi.org/10.1037/10157-006.

———. *Evaluating Competencies: Forensic Assessments and Instruments.* 2nd ed. New York: Plenum Press, 2003.

Grisso, T., and P. S. Appelbaum. *Assessing Competence to Consent to Treatment: A Guide for Physicians and Other Health Care Professionals.* New York: Oxford University Press, 1998.

Grisso, T., P. S. Appelbaum, and C. Hill-Fotouhi. "The MacCAT-T: A Clinical Tool to Assess Patients' Capacities to Make Treatment Decisions." *Psychiatric Services* 48, no. 11 (1997): 1415–19. http://dx.doi.org/10.1176/ps.48.11.1415.

Gruetzner, H. *Alzheimer's: A Caregiver's Guide and Sourcebook.* New York: Wiley, 1988.

Gupta, A., and C. Iadecola. "Impaired Aβ Clearance: A Potential Link Between Atherosclerosis and Alzheimer's Disease." *Name: Frontiers in Aging Neuroscience* 7 (2015): 115. http://dx.doi.org/10.3389/fnagi.2015.00115.

Gurman, A. S., and D. P. Kriskern, eds. *Handbook of Family Therapy,* vol. 2. New York: Taylor and Francis, 1991.

Hachinski, V. C. "Differential Diagnosis of Alzheimer's Dementia: Multiinfarct Dementia." In *Alzheimer's Disease: The Standard Reference,* edited by B. Reisberg, 188–92. New York: Free Press, 1983.

Heaton, R. K., G. J. Chelune, J. L. Talley, G. C. Kay, and G. Curtis. *Wisconsin Card Sorting Test Manual,* revised and expanded. Odessa, FL: Psychological Assessment Resources, 1993.

Henry J. Kaiser Family Foundation. "Life Expectancy at Birth (in Years), By Race/Ethnicity." (2015). http://kff.org/other/state-indicator/life-expectancy-by-re/.

Hook, M. *Gentle Exercises and Movement for Frail People.* Plainview, NY: Wellness Reproductions.

Inouye, S. K., C. H. van Dyck, C. A. Alessi, S. Balkin, A. P. Siegal, and R. I. Horwitz. "Clarifying Confusion: The Confusion Assessment Method: A New Method for Detection of Delirium." *Annals of Internal Medicine* 113 (1990): 941–48. http://dx.doi.org/10.7326/0003-4819-113-12-941.

Iverson, D., G. Gronseth, M. Reger, S. Classen, R. Dubinsky, and M. Rizzo. "Practice Parameter Update: Evaluation and Management of Driving Risk in Dementia—Report of the Quality Standards Subcommittee of the American Academy of Neurology." *Neurology* 74 (2010): 1316–24. http://dx.doi.org/10.1212/WNL.0b013e3181da3b0f.

Janofsky, J. S., R. J. McCarthy, and M. F. Folstein. "The Hopkins Competency Assessment Test: A Brief Method for Evaluating Patients' Capacity to Give Informed Consent." *Hospital and Community Psychiatry* 43 (1992): 132–35. http://dx.doi.org/10.1176/ps.43.2.132.

Jost, B. C., and G. T. Grossberg. "The Evolution of Psychiatric Symptoms in Alzheimer's Disease: A Natural History Study." *Journal of the American Geriatrics Society* 44, no. 9 (1996): 1078–81.

Kan, M. J., J. G. Wilson, A. L. Everhart, C. M. Brown, A. N. Hoofnagle, M. Jansen, M. P. Vitek, M. D. Gunn, and Colton, C. A. "Arginine Deprivation and Immune Suppression in a Mouse Model of Alzheimer's Disease." *Journal of Neuroscience* 35 (2015): 5969–82. http://dx.doi.org/10.1523/JNEUROSCI.4668-14.2015.

Kaplan, E. F., H. Goodglass, and S. Weintraub. *The Boston Naming Test.* 2nd ed. Philadelphia: Lea and Febiger, 1983.

Kaplan, H. I., and B. J. Saddock, eds. *Synopsis of Psychiatry.* Baltimore, MD: Williams and Wilkins, 1994.

Kapp, M. B. 1996. "Assessment of Competence to Make Medical Decisions." In *The Practical Handbook of Clinical Gerontology,* edited by L. L. Carstensen, B. A. Edelstein, and L. Dornbrand, 174–87. Thousand Oaks, CA: Sage.

Karp, N., and E. F. Wood. "Guardianship Monitoring: A National Survey of Court Practices." *Stetson Law Review* 37 (2007): 143.

Kaszniak, A. W. "Neuropsychological Consultation to Geriatricians: Issues in the Assessment of Memory Complaints." *Archives of General Psychiatry* 32 (1987): 1569–73. http://dx.doi.org/10.1080/13854048708520034.

————. "Psychological Assessment of the Aging Individual." In *Handbook of the Psychology of Aging,* edited by J. E. Birren and K. W. Schaie, 427–45. 3rd ed. San Diego: Academic Press, 1990. http://dx.doi.org/10.1016/B978-0-12-101280-9.50031-0.

Kaszniak, A. W., and G. D. Christenson. "Differential Diagnosis of Dementia and Depression." In *Neuropsychological Assessment of Dementia and Depression in Older Adults,* edited by M. Storandt and G. R. Vandenbos, 81–118. Washington, DC: American Psychological Association, 1998.

Kaszniak, A. W., M. Saden, and L. Z. Stern. "Differentiating Depression from Organic Brain Syndromes in Older Age." In *Depression in the Elderly: An Interdisciplinary Approach,* edited by G. M. Chaisson-Stewart, 161–89. New York: Wiley, 1985.

Katz, L. C., and M. Rubin. *Keep Your Brain Alive: 83 Neurobic Exercises to Help Prevent Memory Loss and Increase Mental Fitness.* New York: Workman, 1999.

Kelley, A. S., K. McGarry, R. Gorges, and J. S. Skinner. "The Burden of Health Care Costs for Patients with Dementia in the Last 5 Years of Life." *Annals of Internal Medicine* 163 (2015): 729–36. http://dx.doi.org/10.7326/M15-0381.

Kemp, B. J., and J. M. Mitchell. "Functional Assessment in Geriatric Mental Health." In *Handbook of Mental Health and Aging,* edited by J. E. Birren, R. B. Sloan, and G. D. Cohen, 671–97. San Diego: Academic Press, 1992. http://dx.doi.org/10.1016/B978-0-12-101277-9.50028-0.

Kidd, P. M. "A Review of Nutrients and Botanicals in the Integrative Management of Cognitive Dysfunction." *Alternative Medicine* 3 (1999): 144–61.

Kilada, S., A. Gamaldo, E. A. Grant, A. Moghekar, J. D. Morris, and R. J. O'Brien. "Brief Screening Tests for the Diagnosis of Dementia: Comparison with the Mini-Mental State Exam." *Alzheimer Disease and Associated Disorders* 19 (2005): 8–16. http://dx.doi.org/10.1097/01.wad.0000155381.01350.bf.

Köhler, S., F. Buntinx, K. Palmer, and M. Akker. "Depression, Vascular Factors, and Risk of Dementia in Primary Care: A Retrospective Cohort Study." *Journal of the American Geriatrics Society* 63, no. 4 (2015): 692–98. http://dx.doi.org/10.1111/jgs.13357.

Kornfield, J. *Buddha's Little Instruction Book.* New York: Bantam, 1994.

Koudinov, A. R., and N. V. Koudinova. "Amyloid Beta Protein Restores Hippocampal Long Term Potentiation: A Central Role for Cholesterol?" *Neurobiology of Lipids* 1, no. 8 (2003): 46–56.

La Rue, A. *Aging and Neuropsychological Assessment.* New York: Plenum, 1992. http://dx.doi.org/10.1007/978-1-4757-9119-8.

La Rue, A., C. Dessonville, and L. F. Jarvik. "Aging and Mental Disorders." In *Handbook of the Psychology of Aging,* edited by J. E. Birren and K. W. Schaie, 664–702. 2nd ed. New York: Van Norstrand Reinhold, 1985.

La Rue, A., J. Yang, and S. Osato, "Neuropsychological Assessment." In *Handbook of Mental Health and Aging,* edited by J. E. Birren, R. B. Sloan, and G. D. Cohen, 643–70. San Diego: Academic Press, 1992. http://dx.doi.org/10.1016/B978-0-12 -101277-9.50027-9.

Ladislav, V., D. G. Harper, B. C. Manning, R. Goldstein, R., and A. Satlin. "Sundowning and Circadian Rhythms in Alzheimer's Disease." *American Journal of Psychiatry* 158 (2001): 704–11. http://dx.doi.org/10.1176/appi.ajp.158.5.704.

Larson, E. B., L. Wang, J. D. Bowen, W. C. McCormick, L. Teri, P. Crane, and W. Kukull. "Exercise is Associated with Reduced Risk for Incident Dementia among Persons 65 Years of Age and Older." *Annals of Internal Medicine* 144 (2006): 73–81. http://dx.doi .org/10.7326/0003-4819-144-2-200601170-00004.

Laske, C., H. R. Sohrabi, S. M. Frost, K. López-de-Ipiña, P. Garrard, M. Buscema, J. Dauwels et al. "Innovative Diagnostic Tools for Early Detection of Alzheimer's Disease." *Alzheimer's & Dementia* 11 (2015): 561–78. http://dx.doi.org/10.1016/j.jalz.2014.06.004.

Lerner, H. D. "Psychodynamic Issues." In *Handbook of Clinical Geropsychology,* edited by M. Hersen and V. B. Van Hasselt, 29–50. New York: Plenum, 1998. http://dx.doi .org/10.1007/978-1-4899-0130-9_3.

Lisi, L. B., and S. Barinaga-Burch. "National Study of Guardianship Systems: Summary of Findings and Recommendations." *Clearinghouse Review* 29 (1995): 643.

Liston, E. H. "Diagnosis and Management of Delirium in the Elderly Patient." *Psychiatric Annals* 14 (1984): 117. http://dx.doi.org/10.3928/0048-5713-19840201-07.

Locascio, J. J., J. H. Growdon, and S. Corkin. "Cognitive Test Performance in Detecting, Staging, and Tracking Alzheimer's Disease." *Archives of Neurology* 52 (1995): 1087–99. http://dx.doi.org/10.1001/archneur.1995.00540350081020.

Loewenstein, D., E. Amigo, R. Duara, A. Guterman, D. Hurwitz et al. "A New Scale for the Assessment of Functional Status in Alzheimer's and Related Disorders." *Journal of Gerontology* 44 (1989): 114–21. http://dx.doi.org/10.1093/geronj/44.4.P114.

Logsdon, R. G., and L. Teri. "Identifying Pleasant Activities for Alzheimer's Patients: The Pleasant Events Schedule–AD." *Gerontologist* 31 (1991): 124–27. http://dx.doi .org/10.1093/geront/31.1.124.

———. "The Pleasant Events Schedule–AD." *Gerontologist* 37 (1997): 40–45. http:// dx.doi.org/10.1093/geront/37.1.40.

Lyketsos, C. G. "Current Issues in Dementia Care." *Audio Digest Psychiatry* 33, no. 18 (2004).

Mace, N. L., and P. V. Rabins. *The 36-Hour Day.* Baltimore, MD: Johns Hopkins University Press, 1996.

Marcello, E., F. Gardoni, and M. Di Luca. "Alzheimer's Disease and Modern Lifestyle: What is the Role of Stress?" *Journal of Neurochemistry* 134, no. 5 (2015): 795–98. http://dx.doi.org/10.1111/jnc.13210.

Marengo, J., and J. F. Westermeyer. "Schizophrenia and Delusional Disorder." In *The Practical Handbook of Clinical Gerontology,* edited by L. L. Carstensen, B. A. Edelstein, and L. Dornbrand, 255–73. Thousand Oaks, CA: Sage, 1996.

Markin, R. E. *The Alzheimer's Cope Book: The Complete Care Manual for Patients and Their Families.* New York: Citadel Press, 1992.

Mast, B. T., B. Yochim, S. E. MacNeil, and P. A. Lichtenberg. "Risk Factors for Geriatric Depression: The Importance of Executive Functioning within the Vascular Depression Hypothesis." *Journals of Gerontology Series A: Biological Sciences and Medical Sciences* 59 (2004): 1290–94. http://dx.doi.org/10.1093/gerona/59.12.1290.

Mattis, S. *The Dementia Rating Scale.* Odessa, FL: Psychological Assessment Resources, 2001.

Mayeux, R., and M. Sano. "Drug Therapy: Treatment of Alzheimer's Disease." *New England Journal of Medicine* 341 (1999): 1670–79. http://dx.doi.org/10.1056/NEJM 199911253412207.

McBride, C. M. "Personal Genomic Tests for Healthy Aging: Neither Feast nor Foul." *Generations* 39, no. 1 (2015): 41.

McClure, R., D. Yanagisawa, D. Stec, D. Abdollahian, D. Koktysh, D. Xhillari, R. Jaeger et al. "Inhalable Curcumin: Offering the Potential for Translation to Imaging and Treatment of Alzheimer's Disease." *Journal of Alzheimer's Disease* 44 (2015): 283–95. http://dx.doi.org/10.3233/JAD-140798.

McConnell, L. M., B. A. Koenig, R. T. Greely, and T. A. Raffin. "Genetic Testing and Alzheimer Disease: Recommendations of the Stanford Program in Genomics, Ethics, and Society." *Genetic Testing* 3 (1999): 3–12. http://dx.doi.org/10.1089/gte.1999.3.3.

Meinzer M., R. Lindenberg, M. T. Phan, L. Ulm, C. Volk, and A. Flöel "Transcranial Direct Current Stimulation in Mild Cognitive Impairment: Behavioral Effects and Neural Mechanisms." *Alzheimer's & Dementia* 11 (2015): 1032–40. http://dx.doi .org/10.1016/j.jalz.2014.07.159.

Melton, G. B., J. Petrila, N. G. Poythress, and C. Slobogin. *Psychological Evaluations for the Courts: A Handbook for Mental Health Professionals and Lawyers.* New York: Guilford Press, 2007.

Miguel-Álvarez, M., Santos-Lozano, A., Sanchis-Gomar, F., Fiuza-Luces, C., Pareja-Galeano, H., Garatachea, N., and Lucia, A. Non-steroidal Anti-inflammatory Drugs as a Treatment for Alzheimer's Disease: A Systematic Review and Meta-analysis of Treatment Effect. *Drugs & Aging* 32 (2015): 139–47. http://dx.doi.org/10.1007/s40266-015-0239-z.

Miles, T. P., T. E. Froehlich, S. T. Bogardus, and S. K. Inouye. "Dementia and Race:

Are There Differences Between African Americans and Caucasians?" *Journal of the American Geriatrics Society* 49 (2001): 477–84. http://dx.doi.org/10.1046/j.1532-5415.2001.49096.x.

Miller, M. D., and R. L. Silberman. "Using Interpersonal Psychotherapy with Depressed Elders." In *A Guide to Psychotherapy and Aging,* edited by S. H. Zarit and B. G. Knight, 83–99. Washington, DC: American Psychological Association Press, 1996. http://dx.doi.org/10.1037/10211-003.

Morris, M. C., C. C. Tangney, Y. Wang, F. M. Sacks, D. A. Bennett, and N. T. Aggarwal. "MIND Diet Associated with Reduced Incidence of Alzheimer's Disease." *Alzheimer's Dementia* 11 (2015): 1007–14. http://dx.doi.org/10.1016/j.jalz.2014.11.009.

Moye, J. "Guardianship and Conservatorship." In *Evaluating Competencies: Forensic Assessments and Instruments,* 2nd ed., edited by T. Grisso, 309–89. New York: Springer, 2003.

Moye, J., D. C. Marson, and B. Edelstein. "Assessment of Capacity in an Aging Society." *American Psychologist* 68, no. 3 (2013): 158–71. http://dx.doi.org/10.1037/a0032159.

Moye, J., M. J. Karel, B. Edelstein, B. Hicken, J. C. Armesto, and R. J. Gurrera. "Assessment of Capacity to Consent to Treatment" *Clinical Gerontologist* 31 (2007): 37–66.

Mulsant, B. H., and J. Rosen, "Dementia (Alzheimer's Disease)," in *Handbook of Prescriptive Treatments for Adults,* edited by M. Hersen and R. T. Ammerman, 31–51. New York: Plenum, 1994. http://dx.doi.org/10.1007/978-1-4899-1456-9_2.

Naoi, M., P. Riederer, and W. Maruyama. "Modulation of Monoamine Oxidase (MAO) Expression in Neuropsychiatric Disorders: Genetic and Environmental Factors Involved in Type A MAO Expression." *Journal of Neural Transmission* 123, no. 2 (2016): 91–106. http://dx.doi.org/10.1007/s00702-014-1362-4.

Nasreddine, Z. S., N. A. Phillips, V. Bédirian, S. Charbonneau, V. Whitehead, I. Collin, J. L. Cummings, and H. Chertkow. "The Montreal Cognitive Assessment, MoCA: A Brief Screening Tool for Mild Cognitive Impairment." *Journal of the American Geriatric Society* 53, No. 4 (2005): 695–99. http://dx.doi.org/10.1111/j.1532-5415.2005.53221.x.

Needels, T., and T. Bilanow. "Power Up Your Brain." *Psychology Today,* July 1, 2002, 44–51.

Nekola, P. *An Alzheimer's Guide: Activities and Issues for People Who Care.* Waukesha, WI: Applewood Ink, 2002.

Olsson, R., R. Kucharewski, and H. Eichner. "The Reality Comprehension Clock Test: A Validity Analysis." *Expanding Horizons in Therapeutic Recreation* 19 (2001): 128–32.

Packer, L., and C. Colman. *The Antioxidant Miracle: Your Complete Plan for Total Health.* New York: Wiley, 1999.

Pajeau, A. K., and G. C. Roman. "HIV Encephalopathy and Dementia." In *The Psychiatric Clinics of North America: The Interface of Psychiatry and Neurology,* vol. 15, edited by J. Biller, and R. G. Kathol, 455–66. Philadelphia: Saunders, 1992.

Pan, C., A. Korff, D. Galasko, C. Ginghina, E. Peskind, G. Li, G., T. J. Montine. "Diagnostic Values of Cerebrospinal Fluid T-Tau and Aβ42 Using Meso Scale Discovery Assays for Alzheimer's Disease." *Journal of Alzheimer's Disease* 45, no. 3 (2015): 709–19.

Pearlson, G., and P. Rabins. "The Late Onset Psychosis: Possible Risk Factors." *Psychiatric Clinics of North America* 11 (1988): 15–32.

Petersen, R., ed. *Mayo Clinic on Alzheimer's Disease.* Rochester, MN: Mayo Clinic Health Information, 2002.

Phillips, M. A., C. E. Childs, P. C. Calder, and P. J. Rogers. "No Effect of Omega-3 Fatty Acid Supplementation on Cognition and Mood in Individuals with Cognitive Impairment and Probable Alzheimer's Disease: A Randomised Controlled Trial." *International Journal of Molecular Sciences* 16, no. 10 (2015): 24600–24613. http://dx.doi.org/10.3390/ijms161024600.

Powell, L. S., and K. Courtice. *Alzheimer's Disease: A Guide for Families and Caregivers.* Cambridge, MA: Perseus, 2002.

Qaseem, A., V. Snow, J. T. Cross, M. A. Forciea, R. Hopkins, P. Shekelle, A. Adelman et al. "Current Pharmacologic Treatment of Dementia: a Clinical Practice Guideline from the American College of Physicians and the American Academy of Family Physicians." *Annals of Internal Medicine* 148 (2008): 370–78. http://dx.doi.org/10.7326/0003-4819 -148-5-200803040-00008.

Rama Krishnan, K. R. "Vascular Disease and Depression." *Audio Digest Psychiatry* 34, no. 1. (2005).

Ramanan, V. K., S. L. Risacher, K. Nho, S. Kim, L. Shen, B. C. McDonald, K. K. Yoder et al. "GWAS of Longitudinal Amyloid Accumulation on 18F-florbetapir PET in Alzheimer's Disease Implicates Microglial Activation Gene IL1RAP." *Brain* 138 (2015): 3076–88. http://dx.doi.org/10.1093/brain/awv231.

Ramírez, B. G., C. Blázquez, T. Gómez del Pulgar, M. Guzmán, and M. L. de Ceballos. "Prevention of Alzheimer's Disease Pathology by Cannabinoids: Neuroprotection Mediated by Blockade of Microglial Activation." *Journal of Neuroscience* 25 (2005): 1904–13. http://dx.doi.org/10.1523/JNEUROSCI.4540-04.2005.

Raskind, M. A., and E. R. Peskind. "Alzheimer's Disease and Other Dementing Disorders." In *Handbook of Mental Health and Aging,* edited by J. E. Birren, R. B. Sloan, and G. D. Cohen, 477–513. San Diego: Academic Press, 1992. http://dx.doi.org/10.1016 /B978-0-12-101277-9.50022-X.

Regnier, V., and J. Pynoos. "Environmental Intervention for Cognitively Impaired Older Persons." In *Handbook of Mental Health and Aging,* J. E. Birren, R. B. Sloan, and G. D. Cohen, 763–92. San Diego: Academic Press, 1992. http://dx.doi.org/10.1016 /B978-0-12-101277-9.50031-0.

Reisberg, B. "Alzheimer's Disease." In *Comprehensive Review of Geriatric Psychiatry-II,* edited by J. Sadavoy, L. W. Lazarus, L. F. Jarvik, and G. T. Grossberg, 401–58. Washington, DC: American Psychiatric Press, 1996.

Reisberg, B., S. H. Ferris, M. J. de Leon, and T. Crook. "The Global Deterioration Scale for Assessment of Primary Degenerative Dementia." *American Journal of Psychiatry* 139 (1982): 1136–39. http://dx.doi.org/10.1176/ajp.139.9.1136.

Relkin, N. "Clinical Trials of Intravenous Immunoglobulin for Alzheimer's Disease." *Journal of Clinical Immunology* 34, no. 1 (2014): 74–79. http://dx.doi.org/10.1007/s10875-014-0041-4.

Roeber, S., F. Müller-Sarnowski, J. Kress, D. Edbauer, T. Kuhlmann, F. Tüttelmann, C. Schindler et al. "Three Novel Presenilin 1 Mutations Marking the Wide Spectrum of Age at Onset and Clinical Patterns in Familial Alzheimer's Disease." *Journal of Neural Transmission* 122, no. 12 (2015): 1715–19. http://dx.doi.org/10.1007/s00702-015-1450-0.

Rosen, W. G., R. C. Mohs, and K. L. Davis. "A New Rating Scale for Alzheimer's Disease." *American Journal of Psychiatry* 141 (1984): 1356–64. http://dx.doi.org/10.1176/ajp.141.11.1356.

Sahakian, W. S. *Psychotherapy and Counseling: Techniques in Intervention.* Chicago: Rand McNally, 1976.

Satlin, A., L. Volicer, V. Ross, L. Herz, and S. Campbell. "Bright Light Treatment of Behavioral and Sleep Disturbances in Patients with Alzheimer's Disease." *American Journal of Psychiatry* 149 (1992): 1028–32. http://dx.doi.org/10.1176/ajp.149.8.1028.

Scharre, D. W. "Treatment of Dementia." Ohio Medical Education Network. April, 26–29, 1999. Broadcast.

Schmand, B., J. H. Smit, M. I. Geerlings, and J. Lindeboom. "The Effects of Intelligence and Education on the Development of Dementia: A Test of the Brain Reserve Hypothesis." *Psychological Medicine* 27 (1997): 1337–44. http://dx.doi.org/10.1017/S0033291797005461.

Schneider, J. "Geriatric Psychopharmacology." In *The Practical Handbook of Clinical Gerontology,* edited by L. L. Carstensen, B. A. Edelstein, and L. Dornbrand, 481–542. Thousand Oaks, CA: Sage, 1996.

Sharoff, K. *Coping Skills for Managing Chronic and Terminal Illness.* New York: Springer, 2004.

Sheikh, J. I., and J. A. Yesavage. "Geriatric Depression Scale (GDS): Recent Evidence and Development of a Shorter Version." In *Clinical Gerontology: A Guide to Assessment and Intervention,* edited by T. L. Brink, 165–73. New York: Haworth Press, 1988.

Shen, L., and H. F. Ji. "Associations Between Homocysteine, Folic Acid, Vitamin B12 and Alzheimer's Disease: Insights from Meta-Analyses." *Journal of Alzheimer's Disease* 46 no. 3 (2015): 777–90. http://dx.doi.org/10.3233/JAD-150140.

Shumaker, S. A., C. Legault, S. R. Rapp, L. Thal, R. B. Wallace, J. K. Ockene, S. L.

Hendrix et al. "Estrogen Plus Progestin and the Incidence of Dementia and Mild Cognitive Impairment in Postmenopausal Women: The Women's Health Initiative Memory Study—A Randomized Controlled Trial." *Journal of the American Medical Association* 289 (2003): 2651–62. http://dx.doi.org/10.1001/jama.289.20.2651.

Sjögren, M., and K. Blennow. "The Link Between Cholesterol and Alzheimer's Disease." *World Journal of Biological Psychiatry* 6 (2005): 85–97. http://dx.doi .org/10.1080/15622970510029795.

Snowdon, D. *Aging with Grace: What the Nun Study Teaches Us about Leading Longer, Healthier and More Meaningful Lives.* New York: Bantam, 2001.

Snowdon, D. A., S. J. Kemper, and J. A. Mortimer. "Linguistic Ability in Early Life and Cognitive Function and Alzheimer's Disease in Late Life." *Journal of the American Medical Association* 275 (1996): 528–32. http://dx.doi.org/10.1001/jama.1996 .03530310034029.

Steenland, K., F. C. Goldstein, A. Levey, and W. Wharton. "A Meta-Analysis of Alzheimer's Disease Incidence and Prevalence Comparing African-Americans and Caucasians." *Journal of Alzheimer's Disease* 50, no. 1 (2015): 71–76. http://dx.doi.org/10.3233 /JAD-150778.

Storch, A., A. Hermann, R. Gastl, S. Liebau, O. M. Popa et al. "Adult Human Bone Marrow-Derived Neural Stem Cells: A New Cell Source for Neurorestorative Strategies." Paper presented at the 56th Annual Meeting of the Academy of Neurology, San Francisco, CA, April 2004.

Stoudemire, A., and T. L. Thompson. "Recognizing and Treating Dementia." *Geriatrics* 36 (1981): 112.

Strahan, G. W. *An Overview of Nursing Homes and Their Current Residents: Data from the 1995 National Nursing Home Survey.* Hyattsville, MD: U.S. Department of Health and Human Services, 1995.

———. *Mental Illness in Nursing Homes.* Hyattsville, MD: U.S. Department of Health and Human Services, 1985.

Strub, R. C., and F. W. Black. *Neurobehavioral Disorders: A Clinical Approach.* Philadelphia: F. A. Davis, 1988.

Suh, Y.-H., and F. Checler. "Amyloid Precursor Protein, Presenilins, and Alpha-synuclein: Molecular Pathogenesis and Pharmacological Applications in Alzheimer's Disease." *Pharmacological Reviews* 54 (2002): 469–525. http://dx.doi.org/10.1124/pr.54.3.469.

Sulistio, Y. A., and K. Heese. "Proteomics in Traditional Chinese Medicine with an Emphasis on Alzheimer's Disease." *Evidence-Based Complementary and Alternative Medicine* 2015 (2015). http://dx.doi.org/10.1155/2015/393510.

Sullivan, H. S. *The Interpersonal Theory of Psychiatry.* New York: Norton, 1953.

Tariq, S. H., N. Tumosa, J. T. Chibnall, M. Perry III, and J. E. Morley. "Comparison of the Saint Louis University Mental Status Examination and the Mini-Mental State Examination for Detecting Dementia and Mild Neurocognitive Disorder: A Pilot Study." *American Journal of Geriatric Psychiatry* 14, no. 11 (2006): 900–910. http://dx.doi.org/0.1097/01.JGP.0000221510.33817.86.

Taylor, W. D., H. J. Aizenstein, and G. S. Alexopoulos. "The Vascular Depression Hypothesis: Mechanisms Linking Vascular Disease with Depression." *Molecular Psychiatry* 18, no. 9 (2013): 963–74. http://dx.doi.org/10.1038/mp.2013.20.

Teunisse, S., and M. M. A. Derix. "The Interview for Deterioration in Daily Living Activities in Dementia: Agreement Between Primary and Secondary Caregivers." *International Psychogeriatrics* 9 (1997): 155–62. http://dx.doi.org/10.1017/S1041610297004845.

Tsai, J. L., and L. L. Carstensen. "Clinical Intervention with Ethnic Minority Elders." In *The Practical Handbook of Clinical Gerontology* edited by L. L. Carstensen, B. A. Edelstein, and L. Dornbrand, 76–106. Thousand Oaks, CA: Sage, 1996.

Turner, R. S., R. G. Thomas, S. Craft, C. H. van Dyck, J. Mintzer, B. A. Reynolds, J. B. Brewer et al. "A Randomized, Double-Blind, Placebo-Controlled Trial of Resveratrol for Alzheimer Disease." *Neurology* 85 (2015): 1383–91. http://dx.doi.org/10.1212/WNL .0000000000002035.

Underwood, E. Alzheimer's Amyloid Theory Gets Modest Boost. *Science* 349 (2015): 464. http://dx.doi.org/10.1126/science.349.6247.464.

U.S. Department of Health and Human Services. *Dietary Guidelines for Americans.* Washington, DC: U.S. Department of Health and Human Services, 2005.

———. *Mental Health: A Report of the Surgeon General.* Rockville, MD: U.S. Department of Health and Human Services, 1999. https://profiles.nlm.nih.gov/ps/access/NNBBHS.pdf.

Vaillant, G. E. *Aging Well: Surprising Guideposts to a Happier Life from the Landmark Harvard Study of Adult Development.* New York: Little, Brown and Company, 2002.

Velayudhan, L. "Smell Identification Function and Alzheimer's Disease: A Selective Review." *Current Opinion in Psychiatry* 28, no. 2 (2015): 173–79.

Victoroff, J. *Saving Your Brain: The Revolutionary Way to Boost Brain Power, Improve Memory, and Protect Yourself against Aging and Alzheimer's.* New York: Bantam Dell, 2002.

Warner, M. L. *The Complete Guide to Alzheimer's-Proofing Your Home.* West Lafayette, IN: Purdue University Press, 2000.

Wells, C. E. "Pseudodementia." *American Journal of Psychiatry* 136 (1979): 895–900. http://dx.doi.org/10.1176/ajp.136.7.895.

Wechsler, D. *Wechsler Adult Intelligence Scale—III.* San Antonio, TX: The Psychological Corporation, 1997.

———. *Wechsler Memory Scale—III Manual.* San Antonio, TX: The Psychological Corporation, 1997.

Whitbourne, S. K. "Psychological Perspectives on the Normal Aging Process." In *The Practical Handbook of Clinical Gerontology,* edited by L. L. Carstensen, B. A. Edelstein, and L. Dornbrand, 3–35. Thousand Oaks, CA: Sage, 1996.

Wolfe, R., J. Morrow, and B. L. Fredrickson. "Mood Disorders in Older Adults." In *The Practical Handbook of Clinical Gerontology,* L. L. Carstensen, B. A. Edelstein, and L. Dornbrand, 274–303. Thousand Oaks, CA: Sage, 1996.

Wu, S., Y. Ding, F. Wu, R. Li, J. Hou, and P. Mao. "Omega-3 Fatty Acids Intake and Risks of Dementia and Alzheimer's Disease: A Meta-analysis." *Neuroscience & Biobehavioral Reviews* 48 (2015): 1–9. http://dx.doi.org/10.1016/j.neubiorev.2014.11.008.

Youngjohn, J. R., and T. H. Crook. "Dementia." In *The Practical Handbook of Clinical Gerontology,* edited by L. L. Carstensen, B. Edelstein, and L. Dornbrand, 76–106. Thousand Oaks, CA: Sage, 1996.

Yu, J. T., and L. Tan. "Lifestyle Changes Might Prevent Alzheimer's Disease." *Annals of Translational Medicine* 3, no. 15 (2015): 222. http://dx.doi.org/10.3978/j.issn.2305 -5839.2015.09.02.

Zarit, S. H., and B. G. Knight. *A Guide to Psychotherapy and Aging.* Washington, DC: American Psychological Association Press, 1996.

Zonneveld, H. I., E. A. Loehrer, A. Hofman, W. J. Niessen, A. van der Lugt, G. P. Krestin, M. A. Ikram, and Vernooij, M. W., "The Bidirectional Association Between Reduced Cerebral Blood Flow and Brain Atrophy in the General Population." *Journal of Cerebral Blood Flow & Metabolism* 35, no. 11 (2015): 1882–87. http://dx.doi.org/10.1038/jcb-fm.2015.157.

# Index